A LABOR WITH LOVE

A Dad's-to-Be

Guide to

Romance

During

Pregnancy

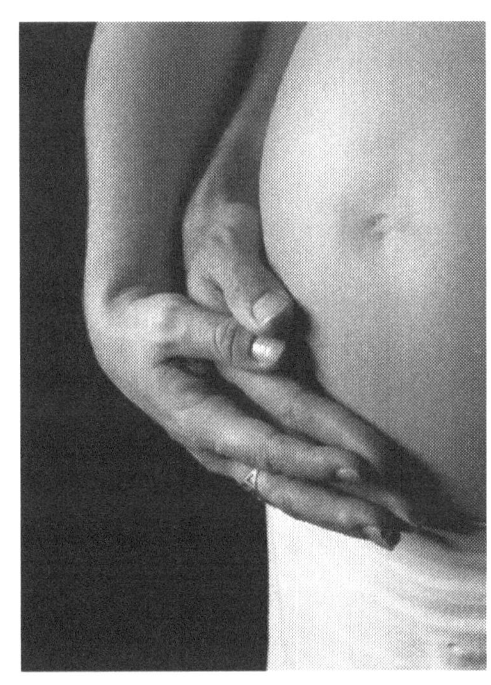

Leon Scott Baxter

A LEWSKI BOOK
Published by Lulu

LEWSKI
Published by Lulu
ISBN 978-1-84728-709-0

Acknowledgments

Writing this book has been an incredible eye-opener for me. I learned more than I had ever anticipated. And, I must thank the one person who inspired me more than any other, my wife of over fourteen years, my best friend and the love of my life, Mary. If it weren't for Mary, I don't think America's Romance Guru would have ever surfaced from my psyche. She has been the inspiration of the romance that has emanated from me over the years. Through Mary's two pregnancies I learned that, to keep the embers of romance alive, I had to change romantically as she changed physically and physiologically. And, she gave me the most precious gifts a man could ever want, our two beautiful girls.

Also, this book would not have been possible without the personal and heartfelt contributions from the moms, new moms, moms-to-be and dads who felt this topic important enough to open their hearts and share their experiences with me and all of the book's readers. I'd like to add special thanks to mother, Allison Stiles, and father, Peter Greenberg, for receiving calls from a complete stranger asking personal questions about their private lives. They offered their stories without hesitation.

Word about the development of *A Labor With Love* was crucial in finding all of the quote contributors. That never would have happened without the support of some phenomenal people, businesses and websites. Two moms who realized the need for this book early on started email chains to their pregnant and new mom friends, as well as women in their Mom-Groups. Thank you so much Rachel Quitner and Ronit Weinstock.

Websites, maternity shops, and other businesses for moms and moms-to-be were integral in getting the word out about the creation of this book as well as displaying and handing out the questionnaires that reaped so many terrific quotes. I'd like to thank AmericanBaby.com, children and infants' store Chicken Little, Kim at Baby Boot Camp, Veronica Melgarejo from Link-upparents.com, Sue Ann Kendall from La Leche League, Rachael Steidl of SantaBarbaraParentSource.com,

Lisa Fell of P.E.P. (as well as all of P.E.P.'s members who participated), Shannon at Due Maternity Shop in Santa Barbara as well as Sydney Lipsky (Due's childbirth instructor).

There were so many folks full of incredible knowledge who didn't think twice when I asked to pick their brains on subjects I was new to. These were personal, intelligent, and helpful professionals. I must thank Catlin Ochse (massage therapist), Jill Dozier (mid-wife), Tracy Schmidt (childbirth educator), Richard F.X. O'Connor (my editor), Juan R. Riker Ph.D. (psychologist) and my agent at Peter Rubie Literary Agency, June Clark, who believed in this book from day one. I can't have an acknowledgments page without thanking my technical advisor and good friend, Marky-Mark Stucky, and the man who pointed me in the right direction for publication, Dr. Don Pedal-Power Lubach.

I feel so fortunate to have had so many people open their mouths, hearts and minds to me. It just allowed me to realize that this subject is one that needed to be approached. I hope their experiences will shed light on some areas of pregnancy, relationships, and romance that may have been in the dark for you, as they have for me.

CONTENTS

A Note To Dads-To-Be

We all remember it. Whether we're dads, grandpas, new fathers, or dads-to-be. Every man who has offered his sperm to create a new life remembers the moment he was told that he was going to be a father. And, I'm no different.

I was pulling into the driveway singing along with the radio, I think it was Cyndi Lauper (it wasn't that this took place so long ago, but it was a Cyndi Lauper song because the station played "the best light sounds from the 80's and 90's."). I hit the garage door opener, and as I pulled in, I saw her. Mary, my wife, was standing there in the garage with this look on her face that I'll never forget. She was smiling, but in an eerie sort of powerful way. It frightened me a bit.

Mary didn't approach the car as I pulled in. She just looked at me. I was a big mouth bass slowly being reeled in by her stare. "What the heck is happening?" I wondered. I turned the car off and jetted out the door.

"What?! What is it? What's going on?"

She continued to hold my eyes with hers. Then, she said the six words that started us on an incredible journey, six unforgettable, simple words:

"You're going to be a daddy."

We'd only started trying two weeks prior. She'd gone to a doctor's appointment earlier that day for a cough she couldn't shake. They gave her a routine pregnancy test, since we'd been trying to conceive, and she passed! A+ first shot. Didn't even have to study. The next thirty-eight weeks were filled with changes and challenges. We learned so much about pregnancy, babies, our relationship and ourselves.

Since that day in 1998, Mary and I have been blessed with two beautiful daughters. It took me six trimesters, eighteen months, two whole pregnancies to realize something, though. See, I'd been in the business of romance for quite some time, giving advice, writing books and articles, holding seminars and such. So, I was pretty aware of my attempts at romance with Mary. I'd try one thing. If it didn't work, I'd try something else until I made my wife happy.

Well, I noticed that during her two pregnancies, I was doing a lot of "searching", trying to find out what made Mary feel special and cared for, what made her feel romanced. As soon as I thought I'd found the trick, Mary would no longer respond to it. So, I'd search some more until I found something else.

This continued throughout her entire first pregnancy. Then, after Baby was born and the dust settled, romance returned to the way it had been during pre-pregnancy days. But, as soon as Mary was pregnant with our second, I was back to the old "hit and miss" romance.

There I was, supposed to be an expert in the field of romance, "America's Romance Guru", and it didn't even dawn on me until after the second baby made her debut, that *romance changes during pregnancy*. Well, at least it did for my wife. So, I started asking around. I spoke with childbirth instructors, ob-gyns, and midwives. Then, I began to question new moms. They all told me that what makes a pregnant woman feel cared for can be a bit different than what worked for her before carrying a child.

I delved deeper, learning about a pregnant woman's physiological changes, as well as what happens to her brain chemistry. And, the pieces were coming together. Yes, it all seemed to make sense. So, I looked for a book to tell me more. What is it precisely that makes a woman feel loved and cared for when pregnant? I couldn't find a single book that could help me. I asked my local librarian. I searched Amazon.com. I walked the aisles of Borders Books. Nothing.

Then, my wife very bluntly asked, "Why don't you write it?"

"Write what?"

"The book you can't find."

"What do you mean?"

"Why don't you find out what it is that men need to know about how to romance their pregnant partners, write it in a book, then, make it available for them to read?'

Sheer genius. She had something there. That's why I married her. I interviewed, questioned, and surveyed hundreds of moms, new moms, and moms-to-be from all walks of life. I spoke with teachers, questioned musicians, surveyed scientists, and interviewed small business owners. These women ranged from pregnant to having thirty-year-old children. They were of diverse ethnic backgrounds, from all across the nation (and a few from Europe), ranging from twenty-one years of age to fifty-five, first-time moms and moms whose hands were full with three or four children.

They all were so pleased to express their opinions on the subject of romance during pregnancy. They shared incredible experiences with me, some filled with pain, others that couldn't help but bring a smile to my face, but all so real, so personal.

I learned more from these women than I had ever anticipated once I started on this journey. This book will be an eye-opener for many men. Because we will never go through pregnancy, there's only so much we can relate to, only so much we can really understand. But, when you hear the same thing from a pregnant twenty-two year old college student, a thirty-four year old teacher and mother of two, as well as a fifty-three year old counselor with kids in college, you've got to sit up and take notice.

So, gentlemen, pay attention! The women tell it to you in their own words in this book. These are our neighbors, our teachers, our doctors, our aunts, our grandmas, and our moms. These are our wives, our partners, our lovers. These are the mothers of our unborn children. Remember, you are where you are today because of the love you shared with the mother of your child. Love created the life she's carrying. Don't let these nine months of changes keep you from showing your partner you love her. Romance will take on a new look for a while. Change with it so your partner can feel that she's cared for by you. You've got a lot riding on this because, "You're going to be a daddy."

Congratulations.

1
Romance Changes During Pregnancy

So, you're going to be a daddy. You must have some ability in the romance department to get this far, but don't send Cupid packing just because your woman is pregnant. On the contrary, romance is all about making your partner feel special, important, and cared for. This is worth repeating, "Romance is making your partner feel special, important and cared for." To each couple, to each individual, this could be manifested in any number of ways: through physical love, kind words, gifts, love letters, compliments, help around the house, a vacation, or a walk on the beach. To offer romance you must know what your partner finds romantic. And, now, more than ever, she needs romance.

During my nearly twenty years of dabbling in the romance field, I've spoken with scores of dads-to-be, many of whom have convoluted ideas with regard to romance during these nine months.

"Oh, she's pregnant, now. She doesn't want all that lovey-dovey stuff. The flowers make her vomit. Her feet are too swollen to go out to dinner. And, she's not going to be interested in any 'evening activities' with a belly that big. She's just too uncomfortable for romance. I'll be romantic again after the baby's born."

WRONG! First mistake, she does want romance. We all do, no matter what state we're in: pregnant, hungry, ecstatic, sleepy, grumpy, or bashful. Remember, romance is making someone feel special, important, and cared for.

Mistake number two is assuming that romance is just flowers, dinner and sex. You have to discover what it is that your partner will find romantic. Romance changes during pregnancy. You must change with it.

And, very likely, the biggest mistake is presuming that if you take a nine-month sabbatical from romance, that you'll be able to jump back in with both feet as soon as Junior is born.

Couples who can't keep the flames of romance burning during pregnancy are going to be left with a bunch of cold, dirty ashes at the end of nine months. And, to think that you'll just pick up where you left off is often very unrealistic for many new parents. A new baby, then toddler, soon-to-be-child, and eventually teen, will zap your time, energy, resources, and libido faster than she can say, "Not tonight, Honey," leaving you with an eighteen year romance hiatus in you relationship. If you don't make it a point to find time for romance, it becomes harder and harder to find time for it after Baby joins the family. So, grab on to the Big R now, and don't let it go.

The problem, I've discovered at my romance seminars, is that many men have difficulty with romance even before pregnancy. Once a man settles into a long-term relationship, romance often packs its bags and heads South for the winter... as well as spring, summer and fall.

But, there is a reason for this (mind you, it's not an excuse). See, Mother Nature wired men and women so that our species would prosper and survive. Men have the ability to sire many children. The more offspring, the better chance that some will survive. Therefore, men are more sexual in nature. Often, when a man is satisfied sexually, he feels as if he's satisfied romantically as well. Why? Dopamine and testosterone levels are high at this time, and a man feels balanced and complete. His brain releases endorphins, neurotransmitters that make him feel happy, energized and motivated. There's no need for anything else (like romance) because he's satisfied, and he assumes, she must be also.

A woman can usually have only one child at a time. Therefore, she's wired to be more emotional, to find a man who will provide and protect her and her offspring. This will better ensure survival of her children as well as herself, allowing her to bear more children and protect those she already has. Therefore, a woman will often feel romanced when she's satisfied emotionally. This emotional satisfaction will increase her oxytocin and serotonin levels leaving her feeling balanced and complete. As a result, her brain releases endorphins, and she feels comforted, delighted, and invigorated.

But, during pregnancy, more than any other time, women's bodies are in tune with nature's survival tactics. The hormones she produces during pregnancy often tell your partner that if you are providing and protecting, if she feels emotionally fulfilled, she's feeling loved.

So, how's a dad-to-be, who may not be a romantic fellow to begin with, supposed to become a master at reading his wife's romantic cravings (which seemingly morph every nineteen minutes) during one of the relationship's most tumultuous experiences... pregnancy? Rub her shoulders. Wash the dishes. Clean up after dinner. You're providing. Talk to the bulge in her belly. Tell her how much you love her and the baby. You're showing signs of protecting. And, that's romance during pregnancy. When she feels provided for, you are meeting her emotional needs, allowing her to reduce her levels of stress and to feel loved.

As you know, things change during pregnancy: energy levels, cravings, body size and shape, intimacy, the home, sleep, and more. But, these changes are normal and should be expected and accepted. The problem for many men is that we don't often realize how extreme the changes can be and how quickly they can take root. Without this knowledge, some men feel compelled to push away from, rather than embrace, the changes and absorb the newness like a good pair of shocks for your four-wheeler.

Susan, a preschool teacher, who contributed her experience for this book, told about her husband's reaction to her pregnancy ten years earlier. He had difficulty absorbing the changes: "I went from thin and active, to gaining weight and exhausted," Susan explained. As a result, "...he actually distanced himself (from me)," finding solace in alcohol, internet pornography, and entertaining younger women. Needless to say, the marriage did not last long after the birth of their child.

Susan's husband's actions were extreme, but the feelings he experienced were not extremely uncommon. The changes going on around him were unexpected and frightening. He reacted by distancing himself from the evolution taking place in his own relationship.

If we, as men, are educated with regard to the changes that may occur during pregnancy, we'll be prepared for them, and thus be more apt to accept them. We'll understand that our lives, our relationships, and our families will be in a state of evolution. Once we accept, understand, and ride out these changes, we've taken the first step, a step that Susan's husband never took. But, this first step is also the easiest in some ways.

Once you can accept and expect the changes, it's time to drop your preconceived notions of romance (if you ever had any in the first place), and start to relearn what romance is all about. What I mean is illustrated during my seminars when I ask men and women to write down what would be most romantic to them. The women often come up with ideas like hot tubbing, going out to dinner, taking a hike or a picnic, going dancing, sharing a bottle of wine. And, the men all nod their heads as if they already do these things.

Well, romance takes on different forms. During courting it could be dancing at a club until 3:00 a.m. It may change to gifts of jewelry during early marriage. After kids, it could be a quiet night with a video. When the kids leave, it may be traveling the continent of Asia. And, when you get to be my grandmother's age, it's a lobster dinner every year on her wedding anniversary. Expect romance to change. And, it will change during pregnancy, too.

The desire for hot tubbing now becomes a desire for a back massage. Taking a hike or picnic becomes taking over the duty of washing clothes. Going dancing is now going to a bed and breakfast. Sharing a bottle of wine is now sharing your feelings, fears, and excitement about the future.

So, how are your going to know exactly what to do and when? Ask. Communicate. The basis of a good relationship is great communication. And, good romance is listening to what your partner is saying and acting in accordance. Know your partner. Talk with her. Read her body language. Use these two questions: "What can I do for you?" and "Do you need anything?" They are like gold. They will get you far during this pregnancy. But, don't stop there. Listen to the answers; then, try and fill her requests.

In many couples the man sees love one way (maybe being told how great a partner he is, or getting a handmade gift), while the woman sees love differently (helping around the house, or snuggling on the couch). Although they both want to express their love for one another, their visions of love differ dramatically? Therefore, neither understands the message the other is trying to convey when they express love the way they "see" love. Gary Chapman wrote a fantastic book on the subject, which I refer to in my seminars called *The Five Love Languages.* You might want to pick it up.

My suggestion: during these nine months, don't rely on what your partner used to find romantic. Nor should you rely on what you find romantic or *think* she'd find romantic. Learn her language of love. Ask her what she wants. Become a bilingual romantic!

"Why?" a buddy of mine asked. "Why should a soon-to-be dad be spending so much time becoming a 'bilingual romantic'? Shouldn't he be reading up on babies and birthing classes? Shouldn't he be putting together the crib and painting nursery walls or something? Sure, he should make his wife feel comfortable and all, but that's a lot of time wasted on romance if you ask me. Why invest so much time on romance?"

Great question. There's a great answer for it, too. Romancing your pregnant wife not only makes her feel good, but it benefits soon-to-be Pop, too. When a man has romanced his partner, he feels as though he's completed a task, a chore that increases the levels of dopamine and testosterone in his brain. This releases endorphins in the brain, which makes us feel absolutely fantastic! With this increase in testosterone and release of endorphins, as well as dopamine, men become more efficient at work. We're energized and motivated. We exercise more, as well as sleep better. Our attention spans increase and stress levels decrease. We're also more able to tolerate the intolerable.

Imagine how life will be at this house: a pregnant woman feeling loved and cared for, her mind at ease. She feels protected and loved during one of the most vulnerable times in her life. And, a man who's rolling with the changes and surprises life lies before him. He's staying fit, sleeping well, is efficient at home and work, able to focus, and when the world seems to be a spinning tornado like the Tasmanian Devil after a double latte, he's level-headed, stress-free, and able to handle almost any obstacle placed in his path.

What a wonderful pregnancy experience this will be. What a harmonious and balanced relationship in which to bring a new life. This is what we'll strive for in this book. And, as we do, you'll come across ideas for different scenarios, but please keep in mind that not everything in this book (or any book on romance) works for every person. Know your partner and communicate.

2
Which Dad-To-Be Are You?

Before we delve too deeply into this sea of "how to romance your pregnant partner", it might behoove you to understand the kind of dad-to-be you're becoming before you jump in with both feet. Although no one man can be pinpointed exactly, to some degree most men fall into one, or more, of the following six variations of expecting fathers.

Take the quiz below, and answer the questions honestly about yourself. Then, see if you agree with the label (or labels) you're slapped with.

The Dads-to-Be Quiz

1. How has your sexual desire changed since the pregnancy?
   A. I can't get enough of her.
   B. No change.
   C. It's dropped faster than Al Roker's weight after his stomach stapling.

2. How would you describe the physical changes in your partner?
   A. She's radiant and glowing.
   B. She's rounder and not much else.
   C. She's fat and clumsy.

3. Finish the following sentence: I can't keep my hands off...
   A. my partner's belly.
   B. the dirty dishes.
   C. the remote control.

4. Which statement sounds most like you?
>   A. I can't wait until the pregnancy is over. I just want my wife back and want to meet my child.
>   B. I can wait as long as it takes. I'm not the one pregnant.
>   C. If she was in a state of perpetual pregnancy, I'd be as pleased as a tomcat at Fisherman's Wharf.

5. Finish this sentence: A man's job in this process is...
>   A. to stay out of the way and let the woman do her thing. Mother Nature knows what she's doing.
>   B. to be available when she asks for something.
>   C. to anticipate her needs and be there for her so she doesn't have to ask for anything.

6. When she starts talking to you about the pregnancy, the birth and how she and the baby are changing you...
>   A. suddenly realize you need to deep clean the microwave oven, get up, and leave.
>   B. turn down the TV and pretend you're listening to her.
>   C. ask questions, because you know you'll never experience pregnancy nor give birth.

7. What is your wife's ob-gyn's name?
>   A. I can say and spell the doctor's name, and know the office phone number by heart.
>   B. I think I got some of the letters right.
>   C. I know it's "Dr. Something".

8. How do you know about the changes taking place with Mom and Baby?
>   A. I read about them in the pregnancy books and magazines, and listen intently at the birthing classes.
>   B. My partner tells me.
>   C. What changes?

9. On a scale of 1 to 10, how would you rate your level of interest in this pregnancy?
       A. 10 ("This is amazing. I'm learning so much.")
       B. 6 ("This is cool.")
       C. 2 ("Down in front. Can't see the game.")

10. When your partner experiences morning sickness, you...
       A. are hugging the Porcelain Goddess in bathroom number two. You just can't take it.
       B. hand her a towel and a toothbrush when she's done.
       C. hold her hair to the side and rub her back, despite the sight and smell.

11. If your partner's water breaks on the kitchen floor...
       A. she'll have to clean it when she gets back home. You won't come within ten feet of that mess.
       B. you'll first cover yourself from head to toe in latex, then clean it up.
       C. no biggie. You'll just clean it up and be on your way to the delivery.

12. The thought of you actually witnessing the birth of your baby...
       A. is enough to get you lightheaded, gives you reason to keep your eyes shut during delivery, and stop you from ever procreating again.
       B. makes you a little queasy, but not enough to scare you away from the delivery room.
       C. is something you've been looking forward to for quite some time.

13. Which phrase do you find yourself saying most to your partner?
       A. "What can I do for you?"
       B. "Where's my green shirt?"
       C. "Can you get me a beer while you're up?"

14. When you touch your partner most often, what's the reason?
    A. To give her a back rub or foot massage.
    B. To smack her behind as she passes in front of the TV.
    C. To have her give you a hand as you try to get up from the sofa.

15. How's the house look since the pregnancy?
    A. Great. I've taken up the slack for my partner.
    B. It's a pigsty. She's let everything fall apart.
    C. Great. She's really kicked it into high gear, even with the edema and hemorrhoids.

16. How do you generally deal with change in your life (at home, at work, etc...)?
    A. I resist it like a stubborn mule.
    B. I roll with the punches.
    C. I embrace change and even seek it out, because change allows me to grow as an individual.

17. When you look to the future, after Baby is born, what TV show are you starring in?
    A. *Married With Children* (financial struggles and a stressed relationship with your partner)
    B. *The Wonder Years* (some ups and some downs)
    C. *Leave It to Beaver* (the perfect American family)

18. When I think about myself as a dad for the rest of my life...
    A. I'm worried for my kid.
    B. I think I'll learn as I go.
    C. I can't wait to start.

Scoring

Next to each number, write down your answer letter. Give yourself three points for every A. B's are worth two points, and C's are one. Total the first three questions (questions 1, 2, and 3). Then, total your next three questions (numbers 4, 5, and 6). Continue in this manner until you've totaled all eighteen questions and have 6 separate totals.

	1.	10.	
	2.	11.	
Total	3.	12.	Total
	4.	13.	
	5.	14.	
Total	6.	15.	Total
	7.	16.	
	8.	17.	
Total	9.	18.	Total

What Do The Scores Mean?

Most men do not fall exclusively into one "Dad-to-Be" category. We may be a little of this, a lot of that, and none of the other. But, this short quiz will allow you to see with which type (or types) of dads-to-be you might identify.

If you score an 8 or 9 in a category, there's a good chance this is you. If your score falls in the 5, 6, or 7 range, you may identify with this category a bit, but it's not all encompassing. A score of a 3 or 4 tells you that this really isn't you.

Category #1 - Delighted Dad (Questions 1 - 3)

If you scored an 8 or 9, you are definitely a delighted dad. This whole experience is just incredible for you.

Score a 5, 6, or 7, you're probably enjoying the pregnancy, but it's not something you're jumping up and down about and keeping track of in your daily "daddy diary."

If you scored a 3 or 4, you're really not enjoying this experience. You can't wait until it's over. You actually may identify yourself more as a Fearful Father or a Bystander.

MORE ABOUT DELIGHTED DADS

"I was very physically attracted to my wife. It was like having a new woman every two weeks. I liked the variety."
-R. M., Brand New Father

The Delighted Dad just loves this pregnancy. He feels it brings him closer to his partner. He relishes her changes and looks forward to what the coming weeks have in store. Delighted Dad is very attracted to his partner. He may find the thought of the two of them having created a new life through love a miraculous event, and has become more attracted to his partner on an emotional level.

He may find her new and ever-changing body a physical attraction. Many a Delighted Dad have described their partner's growing body as voluptuous and exciting. He loves the new curves, the big belly, and the rounder breasts.

And, of course, there are Delighted Dads who become more attracted to their partners both emotionally as well as physically. But, one thing they all seem to have in common is that they see their partners as beautiful and radiant. This is usually manifested via compliments and a lot of touching, Most pregnant women will respond favorably to this by producing the hormone oxytocin which leads to endorphins being released in the brain making them feel loved and cared for.

"I looked at her like, 'Wow!' even fifty pounds bigger. I don't know how to explain it. I felt like, 'Man, she's having my kid.' I adored her even more."
-E. W., Loan Officer

Category #2 - Bystander (Questions 4 - 6)

If you scored an 8 or 9, you see yourself more of a Bystander in this pregnancy and less of a participant.

A score of 5, 6, or 7 tells you that you'll get involved, but more because you feel it's your obligation or because she requests it, and less because you really want to be a part of this experience.

If your total was 3 or 4, you've decided not to watch from the sidelines. You're right in there with the action. You may actually be more of a Delighted Dad, Personal Assistant, or an Active Participant.

MORE ABOUT THE BYSTANDER

"I remember, it was hard watching her body change so drastically. It meant the end of us being a couple. There were lots of times when I missed her. There was no sex for months. Sometimes it felt like I only had sex with her to let her know she was attractive and that I loved her, not because we wanted to romp in the hay."
-Mark, Santa Barbara, CA

The Bystander is like Prissy from *Gone With the Wind*: "I don't know noting about birthin' no babies," and I don't care to know about it, neither. The Bystander is a bit standoffish. He removes himself from anything "pregnancy". He may feel as though he's just not comfortable with the entire process: "My father didn't really participate, and my mom was fine with it... It's not a man thing... If God wanted me to get involved, he would have let men carry the babies."

Some men are Bystanders merely because they believe that's what would benefit their partner most: "I don't want to get in her way... She probably won't feel comfortable with me around... This is pretty private stuff. I don't want to embarrass her."

Regardless of the reason, the Bystander is not participating much in his partner's pregnancy. Often he doesn't want to hear about the pregnancy, he won't read about it, and he definitely doesn't want any visual aids. The Bystander endures the pregnancy, rather than relishes the experience, because he knows he'll have a baby at the end of nine months. He's thinking, "Let's get this thing over with. I want to see the baby and just get my wife back."

Many partners of the Bystanders feel abandoned having to fend for themselves during a time that can truly bring couples so much closer. Although some women with traditional, "old school" values may feel a man's place is anywhere but the ob-gyn's office or a delivery room, they too must experience this event alone, not realizing that it can be shared lovingly by two.

If the Bystander steps up, rather than aside, not only is he supporting his wife, but he doesn't have to wait nine months to "get her back". She'll be with him in all her radiant roundness the entire time.

"I missed her. She was really tired and really sick so I left her to herself. She slept so much. I felt alone, by myself."
-Matthew, Elementary School Teacher

Category #3 - Active Participant (Questions 7 - 9)

If your total was an 8 or 9, you've been very much an Active Participant in this pregnancy. You're right there with Mom every step of the way, sharing her experiences and learning as she does.

Score a 5, 6, or 7, and you're a bit more complacent when it comes to the pregnancy. You let it come to you rather than seeking it out yourself. But, once it's there in front of you, you're definitely interested.

A score of 3 or 4 tells you that you haven't participated much in this pregnancy. You may find yourself thinking that this is a woman's experience, not a man's. If so, you may identify more with the Bystander.

MORE ABOUT THE ACTIVE PARTICIPANT

"I'm one of those guys who went to every appointment. We did the natural childbirth classes together. I coached her nutrition-wise,

exercise-wise, and I did it with her. I videotaped her along the way. Her water broke, and I was behind her with a camera."
-Elvin, Father of Two

The man labeled with the title of "Active Participant" will usually remain on his partner's good side during pregnancy. The Active Participant is fully involved with the pregnancy through thick and thicker. Not being able to experience pregnancy firsthand, the Active Participant researches it and learns all he can. He'll read the baby books, subscribe to the pregnancy magazines, spend hours on fetus development websites, and attend all of his partner's ob-gyn appointments.

The Active Participant is very often on top of the baby's monthly developmental changes and the phases Mom is enduring during her trimesters. The entire process of creating a new life intrigues him, how the cells become a real person, and how Mom's body is a vessel for this metamorphosis.

The Active Participant is very supportive of his pregnant partner. He helps her stay healthy by going on walks with her, cooking healthy meals together, and steering clear of cigarettes, alcohol and other potentially dangerous substances.

Most moms would kill for an Active Participant for a partner. But, that's not always the case. Some women prefer to not have their partners so involved. Sometimes it's a matter of modesty; other times it's privacy. Some moms-to-be feel as though it's their right as women to choose how they will experience their pregnancy. And, some men can get a bit too involved, living for the next doctor visit, and putting Mom's trimesters and baby's development at the center of their world.

But, for the most part, an Active Participant will make his partner feel very special, very cared for, and definitely romanced.

"I was very much involved in our pregnancy. I stopped smoking and drinking and we both got into shape. I went to every single doctor's appointment. I made it as much of a priority for me as it was for her. I volunteered to get her vitamins and her food cravings. We had gone

into this together, but she had to do all the hard work. So emotionally, I supported her. A pregnant woman is always right, especially when she's my wife."

-Paul G., Toronto, Canada

Category #4 - Mr. Squeamish (Questions 10 - 12)

For whatever reason, even some of the toughest, burliest of men feel a bit woozy with all of the bodily fluids that come with pregnancy. If you scored an 8 or 9, you may be Mr. Squeamish, a man who feels lightheaded when he envisions the actual delivery and nauseous when his partner has morning sickness.

A 5, 6, or 7, tells you that although a meconium plug and water breaking doesn't make its way into your everyday vernacular, you'll be able to handle them when it's time.

If you scored a 3 or 4, you appear to have your squeamishness under wraps. You know that witnessing the episiotomy or seeing the delivery of the placenta is just another step in this incredible experience. You may be more of a Delighted Dad or an Active Participant.

MORE ABOUT MR. SQUEAMISH

"During our first pregnancy I was definitely uncomfortable during delivery, with all of the blood and the placenta coming out. I was like, 'Holy mackerel!' I felt like passing out."

-Drew, Operations Analyst

Some of us, no matter how supportive we wish to be, just have difficulty with all of the new body fluids that come with pregnancy. It might be the leaky breasts during sex, the morning sickness, or even the water breaking on the front patio. Mr. Squeamish tends to be the man who becomes nauseous at the sight of blood or the thought of the mucous plug.

Most men, squeamish or not, want to be a support for their pregnant partners. But, for a Mr. Squeamish, there's an obstacle keeping him at bay, often when his partner needs him most. Mr.

Squeamish needs to relay his discomforts to his partner, so she will know that it's not her he's staying away from... it's her placenta.

If Dad-to-be and pregnant Mom are okay with this, great. But, if Dad wants to make it through delivery conscious, the two will have to start building up a resistance, desensitizing Dad to pregnancy's less-than-pleasant visuals.

"I was very squeamish about the birth. We went to a birthing class and saw a video on delivery. I was totally squirming and a bit immature about it. I wasn't so sure about the delivery process."
-M. N., Father of Six Month-Old Boy

Category #5 - Personal Assistant (Questions 13 - 15)

With an 8 or 9 in the total box, you are your pregnant partner's Personal Assistant. You realize how much work pregnancy takes and the toll it's taken on her. So, you're doing everything you can to help her out in anyway possible.

If you score a 5, 6, or 7, you're not quite a Personal Assistant, but more of an intern who's on a never-ending coffee break. You haven't changed all that much for her.

With a 3 or 4 you're probably more of a hindrance around the house than a help. You may be in denial about this pregnancy and about what the future holds for you. If so, you may identify more readily with a Fearful Father.

MORE ABOUT THE PERSONAL ASSISTANT

"I did a lot more things to take up the slack and help out more. I made breakfast for her all the time. She loved when I used to squeeze and caress her legs and feet."
-M. S., Father to Ethan, 4, and Jacob, 8

Wouldn't life be great if we all had one, a personal assistant, a person who is there for you, catering to your needs, knowing what you need even before you ask for it? Not all of us can afford an extravagance like this, but some pregnant women find that they have one, nonetheless, in their soon-to-be-dad husbands.

The Personal Assistant's most frequently used phrase is, "What can I do for you?" He is available to help his pregnant partner any way he can. He runs out for her strange food cravings. He gases her car when the tank is half empty. He offers shoulder massages and has become the household chef.

The Personal Assistant doesn't see his partner as helpless so much, but rather sees himself as helpful. He knows she's working hard and struggling through discomforts. So, he chooses to pick up as much slack as possible, so she can focus on having a healthy and stress-free pregnancy.

Most women will be pleased to find their partner fulfilling the role as Personal Assistant. For anyone, it feels wonderful to be catered to. It makes us feel special. That's what spas, gourmet restaurants, flying first class, and five-star resorts are all about. We're pampered and treated as if we are held in high esteem.

But when a woman is pregnant and getting that pampering from the man she loves... without the pricey bill, romance emerges. She feels taken care of because he loves her and her baby. This produces feelings of being protected and looked after, which is safe and nurturing, producing neurotransmitters in the brain that create a euphoric feeling we call romance.

"I tried to do more chores because she could do less. I took on more of the things she'd been doing, like the cooking."
-Elvin, Father of Nathan, 6, and Irelyn, 3

Category #6 - Fearful Father (Questions 16 - 18)

With an 8 or 9 you may be a Fearful father. This pregnancy is uncharted waters for you and you don't do so well with change. The unknown makes you uncomfortable.

If you score a 5, 6, or 7, you are definitely concerned with what the future may hold for you, your relationship and your family. But, you're ready to make due with whatever life has in store for you.

With a 3 or 4 you're really not afraid of the changes you're heading for. You look forward to the challenges and have already told yourself that your future will be bright and full of happiness.

MORE ABOUT FEARFUL FATHER

"It was the life changes. I felt like it was a huge 'growing up thing.' I wasn't ready for it. I felt <u>we</u> weren't ready. I wanted to stay young and be able to do whatever we wanted whenever we wanted. We were going to lose all of that."
-Noel, Age 27

Dads-to-be have fears. New parents have fears. It's common. It's natural. You're venturing into the mysterious unknown. It's exciting, and part of that excitement is the fear of that unknown. But the Fearful Father's fear goes a bit farther than the average Joe. He tends to resist change, not just during this pregnancy, but in life in general: moving to a new office space, eating at a different restaurant, favorite TV show gets canceled, a new guy gives him a haircut. All this irks him.

So, pregnancy really causes stress. That stress is manifested through fear, fear of the weekly changes he sees in his partner, which are insights to life's grander and more drastic changes after baby arrives: "How will we pay for this new person?... What affect will this have on our retirement, investing, and taxes?... What about my relationship with my partner?... Will we both have enough love for the baby and each other?... What about our alone time?... Will I become second fiddle to the baby?... Will there still be time for me?... Can I still go surfing on weekends?... How about watching the games or reading my book each night?... Will my time be sucked up with diaper changing, housecleaning, and baby swaddling?"

Many Fearful Fathers, especially first time dads, are afraid they won't be good enough dads. They're afraid they might "do it wrong", that they'll spoil this untouched life. But this, believe it or not, is a sign of a potentially terrific father. One so concerned about his abilities to father has his intentions in the right place, and that's where parenthood starts, with the right intentions.

Fearful Fathers can't let fear of the future destroy their present if they wish to bring romance to their pregnant partners. Worry doesn't change the future. It merely spoils the present. So, relish this magical time. Prepare for the future, but don't wallow in it. Surround yourself with the magic in front of you, your partner holding the ember of new life. Love her, and let her feel loved.

"I was afraid that after the baby was born, I wouldn't be getting as much attention from my wife as I would like. I also feared the change in her breasts. These things wouldn't be sexual and recreational anymore. They'd have a real use. They would no longer be for me."
-Marcus F., Photographer

One More Thing

Future fathers can fall anywhere on the spectrum of any of the six types of dads-to-be. There's no limit. You can be a full-fledged Mr. Squeamish, Personal Assistant, and Fearful Father all at once. You may identify with maybe one style more than another. It's possible that you'll find that you've got a bit of some of these attributes, but not enough to label you such. What's important here is you starting to analyze yourself as a partner during these nine months.

This pregnancy will happen only once and the memory will last a lifetime. How do you want it to be remembered? How do *you* want to be remembered? If your current actions are leading you to your goal for this pregnancy, capitalize on that. Strengthen what you are doing. Build upon it.

If you're on a path that may lead you to a sour memory of this pregnancy, find a way to make your personality work for you and your partner, for your pregnancy. For example, if you fear that you'll be losing your wife to your baby, and that's distancing you during the pregnancy, tell her. She'll probably be delighted to know she's loved that much by you, that you fear losing her. That, in effect, will bring you closer during pregnancy, which will continue on after Baby arrives.

Remember, we're all different. We come from different backgrounds, have different beliefs, and different expectations. We can't all be the same, and shouldn't. Identify who you are. If you're happy with him, embrace it. If you're not, do something about it. For when you become cognitive of your actions for the one you love, your actions speak love to her. And, although we're all different, there are things we all want for our partners: comfort, happiness and love, which combined, all translate to "romance."

3

The Magic Touch

"Touch!! Massage!! I could never get enough of it. During pregnancy my entire body would ache. Sometimes it was my shoulders, or my back, or my feet, or my legs, and any kind of gentle touch would soothe me."

-Mary L., Mother of Two

Let it be known, this chapter is right up here in front for a very specific reason. If you only get this far in the book, you'll be better off than most ill-prepared dads-to-be. As I conducted research for *A Labor With Love*, I was utterly surprised, pretty much dumbfounded, to find that nearly three out of every four women surveyed, mentioned touch, rubbing, and/or massage in their responses to what they found romantic during pregnancy.

Sure, a massage is always relaxing and can be sensual, and I figured, "I'm sure it's probably soothing during pregnancy." But, not until I spoke with so many women, did I understand the true importance of touch during pregnancy.

Being a man, I couldn't fully appreciate this need for touch while carrying a baby. So, I looked into it to find out why, why more than any other action, touch was mentioned so often.

Most men don't realize that touch can calm Mom-to-be. It can alleviate the common discomforts associated with pregnancy: edema (swollen feet, ankles, and hands), leg cramping, and back pain. Women have reported that massage has helped them fall asleep easier and relieved heartburn as well as morning sickness. Touch can release your woman from the chains of headache, stiff neck, and sciatica (the swelling of the sciatic nerve).

One of the amazing results of touch is that it releases the hormone, oxytocin, in women. Oxytocin has been called the "cuddle chemical". It's the hormone that's released in Mom during breast-feeding, putting her in a calm, relaxing, and loving state.

Your touch can have the same affect on your partner. When the oxytocin levels rise, stress levels decrease. Passion and romance builds. And, she's rewarded with the euphoria of endorphins. In a nutshell, touching her makes your partner feel content and loved on a physiological level, all due to oxytocin, the key to romance.

During these nine months, a pregnant woman's nerve endings are highly sensitive. Find out which areas of her body will be most soothed by your touch, how she likes to be touched there, and then, focus on them.

Each mom-to-be will be different. So, ask. Try a variety of touches, of rubs and strokes, and touch a variety of areas. Read her body language.

The following are the types of touches the surveyed women expressed as most romantic.

Back, Neck & Shoulders

"I would have loved if he'd rubbed my back when I was throwing up in the toilet, and told me to hang in there."
                    - Sue, Preschool Teacher

Women like Sue have said that a rub and a kind word do wonders for them. But, it's not only a rub that many pregnant women crave. Catlin Ochse, a massage therapist who specializes in pregnancy massage, explains that although the general public appreciates neck, shoulder, and back massages, because pregnant women are carrying a heavier load, this type of touch soothes them beyond the average, non-baby-carrying, Joan Public.

It's been advised to avoid deep massage during your partner's first trimester. It could trigger dizziness and morning sickness. But, by the second trimester, she should be ready for your strokes. It's best to massage gently. Remember, pregnant women's bodies are sensitive, and this is not just any pregnant woman. This is your partner. Muscles may be sore; ligaments are being stretched. So, it's best to err on the cautious side. If she needs the rub a bit deeper, she'll tell you.

So, how can you relieve her discomfort? For neck and shoulder massage, sit her in a soft chair where you can reach the intended areas. If you don't have a soft chair, make one. Load up on pillows from your bed, throw pillows from the sofa, or pad her with paper towels and toilet paper rolls, whatever will allow her to relax and enjoy your touches. Or, you could always be seated on the floor, bed or couch leaning back on a support, and your partner can sit between your legs and lean back on your chest.

Let your fingers work their way up and down her neck to the base of her skull. You can gently use your thumb to massage the muscles of her shoulders. This can be done over her clothes or on her bare skin. Use massage oils to reduce friction if you choose, though you may want to avoid aromatherapy oils. Because pregnant women tend to be sensitive to smells; the aroma could result in nausea rather than relaxation.

As for back massage, most doctors don't recommend a pregnant woman lie face down on her belly after the four-month mark. But, that's not an excuse for skimping on a back massage. Your pregnant partner will probably be feeling lots of pressure and strain in her lower back, especially in the later months. Focus here. Have your partner lie on her side, or have her sit leaning forward facing a table or desk loaded with pillows. Then, rub the area around the small of her back. Ask how it feels, then adjust based on what she says.

Ochse advises, "Five minutes makes a huge difference, but one of the biggest complaints I get is that pregnant women's guys will squeeze their shoulders a couple of times and be done, leaving them craving more. Turn off the game. Make the massage intimate. Be present and feel the muscles you hold in your hands."

You can't massage your pregnant partner out of obligation. Why not? Because she will detect this. And, the desired results will not be reached. So, like Ochse recommends, focus on her. It doesn't have to be long. It just has to be about her. Thirty minutes of a back rub while you're on the phone is far less effective that a ten-minute neck rub that's all about her.

"A gentle back massage would have been comforting, especially during the last few months of pregnancy. I feel any contact during the last few months makes you feel good."
                              -Brooke R., Registered Dental Hygienist

Feet & Legs

"A very nice thing he does is rub my feet for me... every night! I'm nine months pregnant and work full time on my feet. I can't think of anything more appreciated than that!"
                              -Sarah G., Professional Musician

Edema, or swelling of the extremities, is very common during pregnancy. Three out of four moms-to-be will experience this discomfort during the end of pregnancy, especially in their feet and hands. Tingling and numbness in your partner's fingers and toes are common due to swelling tissues pressing on the nerves. Because of gravity's pull throughout the day, the discomfort may become more severe in the evening. So, to start, get Mom off her feet, and get them up. Prop her tootsies on a pillow and have her lie back a bit so the fluids can flow away from the swollen parts of her body.

But this, my friend, is only the beginning. You wouldn't believe the number of pregnant women who would do almost anything for a foot rub or a leg massage. Your legs and feet bear the brunt of all the weight, steps and strains you experience on any given day, but when the weight is increasing, the steps are more difficult to take, and the strains are more common than before. Relief through massage is like a gift from heaven.

There are many techniques that you can experiment with and talk to your partner about: oil, slow strokes or deeper tissue massaging. Leg massage can help stimulate blood flow, for many pregnant women experience poor blood circulation through their legs. But, do try to avoid direct massage over varicose veins and swollen areas, which may become apparent during pregnancy. There are many books on the subject of foot and leg massage, as well as books specializing on acupressure and the benefits for pregnant women. Be cautious, though. According to acupressure experts, there are points on both the foot and the lower leg that can induce labor. When I learned of this, I became concerned. What man wants to be the cause of pre-labor contractions? Should men just avoid this part of the body completely?

"No," Ochse assures, "men should not avoid the feet. Instead, avoid deep work and staying in one spot too long. Also, listen to what Mom says works for her. That's always a good rule to go by." Other childbirth experts, as well as moms, maintain that Mom's body will know what's right and what's wrong. Just be sure to listen to your partner, because when asked if the leg and foot massage should be avoided for fear of early labor, not one of the participants were willing to give up the relief. So, go for it, fellas; just do so with mild enthusiasm. (On the same note, if you attempt a hand massage, don't spend much time on the webbing between her thumb and index finger. According to acupressurists this, too, could lead to contractions.)

So, where are the best places to rub on the foot and leg? According to reflexology charts, the foot is like a map of the body. The heel corresponds to the sciatica (the nerve that runs from the lower back down the leg) as well as hemorrhoids. The inside of the heel is attributed to the lower back, whereas the spot on the sole just below the pinky toe is connected to the shoulders. The spot to avoid deep massage is called Spleen 6. It's located on the lower leg, about four fingers above the inner ankle, and can induce labor if massaged deeply for long periods of time.

Don't forget that these touches are soothing, relaxing, and healing, but can also bring you and your partner closer. Touch and massage are not only beneficial for your partner's body, but for your relationship as a couple. When her oxytocin levels rise due to your touch, Mom-to-be suddenly feels the urge to touch you, which increases your oxytocin levels, creating a romantic "touching circle of caring." It is an intimate expression of love.

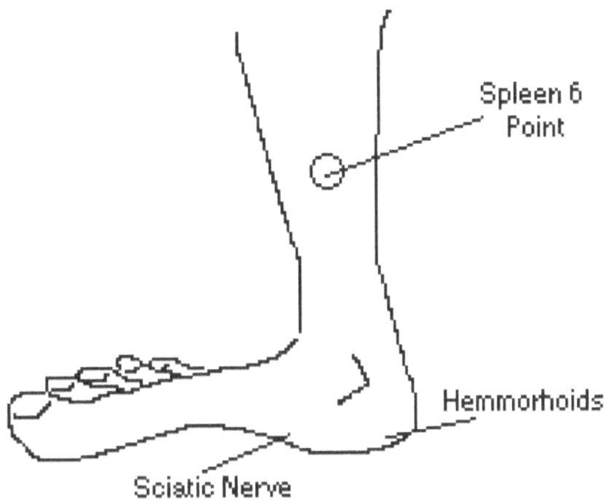

"I would have liked a foot massage. My feet were swollen and tired from carrying my extra load around. It is an extremely intimate and relaxing feeling having someone massage your feet."
-Sancha F., Mother of Two

Belly

"My husband made me feel good when he would rub and massage my belly. I felt good because I felt he was acknowledging me and my unborn baby at the same time, and that was awesome!"
-B.R., Santa Barbara, CA

It's not advisable to actually deep massage your partner's pregnant tummy, but many women find it soothing to have their bellies caressed gently.

Effleurage is a popular technique during labor, but is also very beneficial during pregnancy. As your partner's belly grows, you may notice her subconsciously rubbing the underside of her abdomen as she waits in line at the bank. Or, she may stroke her stomach as she relaxes in front of the TV. The skin of her belly is being stretched and the nerves, again, are very sensitive. Effleurage consists of long gliding strokes (like your partner's already doing for herself) on her belly. With your palm or fingertips follow the underside contours of your partner's abdomen, with a little cornstarch, baby powder, or lotion to reduce friction. This will relax and soothe her as well as connect you to the baby.

But, you don't have to sit down and have an official "effleurage session". Touching your wife's tummy throughout the day will feel good to her and build the bond between you and your unborn baby. Stroke her belly as you pass her in the kitchen. In the bath or shower, lather up her swollen mid-section and give it a gentle, loving cleaning. Walk up behind your partner as she talks on the phone and place your hands on her stomach. Spoon her in bed with your hands resting on the bulge waiting for it to move. Some women love to have oil rubbed on their tummies. Try vitamin E to help reduce friction as well as stretch marks.

Your partner's belly is a very sensitive area, not just because of the heightened nerve endings, but it can also be psychologically sensitive. The growth and change in her body can make her feel unattractive. By giving that growth so much hands-on attention, she'll not only feel soothed physically, but emotionally, as well.

"He sometimes rubbed belly balm onto my belly, which was romantic because it showed how much he liked touching me, even with a large belly."
-Nicole, New Mom

Head

"I would lay on (my husband's) lap while he massaged my head and played with my hair to relax me."
-Debbie, Full-Time Mom

Have you ever been on the receiving end of a thorough scalp massage? If you haven't, you must. Talk about relaxing! It feels as though all the stress that's been built and stored at the base of your head is released through the masseuse's touch, through the skull, up to the scalp, through each hair follicle, and out the fingertips that rub your head. I don't know if a pregnant woman's heightened nerve endings extend to her head, but she certainly is carrying tension in her body, and much of that is stored in the head. A soothing rub can wash away anxiety and allow Mom-to-be to feel romanced.

There are a variety of ways to create this relaxed state of loving, including washing her hair in the shower. Take some time to really rub the shampoo into her scalp. Draw your fingers through her hair several times. Rub the base of her neck with your thumbs.

If you'd like, this can be done in the bathtub (assuming you'll both fit), you leaning against the back of the tub and your pregnant partner leaning lazily against you. Massage therapists say that most people hold an incredible amount of tension around the jaw. Why not try gently rubbing down from the temples along the jaw line and under the cheekbones?

Allow these touches to become touches of love. There's often a unique experience between a pregnant woman and the husband who's massaging her, in comparison to a man massaging the wife who's not pregnant. "I've noticed that there's a different connection," Ochse says, "a unique quality of lovingness that is felt from sharing this special time of pregnancy together."

Even the act of brushing your pregnant partner's hair can be considered soothing, loving, and romantic. You can do it dry or after a bath. Keep in mind, this brushing is not to get the tangles out, nor is it an opportunity to style her quaff. Use it as a connection between you and your partner. Use long strokes through her untangled hair. New mom, Kristy remembers the feeling:

"He used to brush my hair while I laid in his lap, to help me relax toward the end of pregnancy."
-Kristy, Salt Lake City, UT

The Spa Treatment

"Arrange for me to have some sort of spa treatment (e.g. pregnancy massage, pedicure, facial, etc...!). Pampering is so appreciated during pregnancy, and this would be romantic to me because it would show me that he wants me to feel relaxed and cared for."
-L.S., Age 35

So, maybe you're not the most adept at touch and massage. There are scores of books on massage and some focus specifically on prenatal massage. You could read one of these or even take a course on massage. But, if you find that you're still all thumbs, although it's quite a connecting experience between soon-to-be parents, maybe it's time for some professional help.

Even though a licensed massage therapist doesn't necessarily know your partner the way you do, most who've been trained in prenatal massage know what works for pregnant women in general. They know the sensitive spots, the areas that should be avoided, and the points that need more focus. They're familiar with the tenderness of stretching ligaments and know how to position a pregnant woman to maximize her comfort.

Another benefit to hiring a massage therapist is staying power. If you're anything like me, after ten, fifteen minutes max, your hands are pork chops. They become useless, and suddenly I'm the one in dire need of a hand massage. These experts of touch keep going like the Energizer Bunny. Thirty minutes, an hour, an hour and a half, not even a sweat.

If you plan to go the professional route, you might as well look into other methods of pampering by specialists. Maybe make a day of it for your partner. Get her out of the house, and treat her to a day at the spa: facial, massage, mud bath, pedicure, manicure, and the like.

The women surveyed for *A Labor With Love* expressed that they felt romanced not only when their men touched them, but also when they arranged for others to pamper them. A pregnant woman needs a day, now and again, that's not about nurseries and showers and labor-prep, but about her... without you. She gets to have her time and you get to catch the game or take a nap or mow the lawn or read a book. But, when she returns, she'll be relaxed and content, and she'll attribute it all to you.

By the way, fellas, do not let this section be your ticket out of touching your pregnant partner. Just because you arrange a day at the spa or a pregnancy massage, you still need to touch her yourself, and often. It doesn't matter if you can't massage your way out of a wet paper bag. Try. Also, touch that belly; feel your baby kick. Wash your partner in the tub. Brush her hair. There are so many ways to touch your wife without the stress and fear of "massage failure".

"I wish he'd paid for me to get a pregnancy massage."
-Mrs. H., Age 27

Just Touch Her

"In bed he would cuddle me all the time. He was wonderful."
-Rebecca, Manager

As mentioned earlier, you don't have to be a massage therapist to make your partner feel cared for and loved, to make her feel romanced, when it comes to touch. Just touch her on a regular basis. Wrap your arms around that voluptuous woman next to you. Realize that you hold in your arms your partner and the result of your love for her. When you can truly grasp this, your touch can't help but be loving.

We've mentioned ways to express romance through touch: belly caressing, cuddling, brushing and washing her hair, and washing her body. But, what about the simple stuff? Hug the mother of your baby. Hold her hand often, unless, of course, she's not comfortable with it; some women get sweaty palms during pregnancy and need frequent air-drying. Make sure you're in contact with her when you sit on the couch together: knees touching, hand on her leg. Play footsies with her under the dinner table. Touch her because you love her. Let your touches become extensions of that love. You might even try what Lynne hoped her husband would have done to express his love through touch. Strangely, this came up more often than I would have guessed.

"He could have offered to shave my legs for me! This would have been romantic because anytime a man pays that type of careful attention to a woman, it's bound to be sexy and fun. Plus, my legs would have looked so much better if they were smooth."
-Lynne, Associate Director

10 Touch Essentials

1. Offer her a neck rub.
2. Hug her.
3. Give her a lower back massage.
4. Try effleurage.
5. Rub her feet with peppermint foot lotion.
6. Soothe her shoulders with your thumbs as she watches TV.
7. Hire a massage therapist to give her a prenatal massage.
8. Massage her scalp as you wash her hair.
9. Splurge and treat her to a day at the spa.
10. Hold her hand in public.

"He gave me little feet massages, back rubs, looked me in the eyes and asked me, 'How are you, really?'."
-Ellie, Mother of One

4

Make It Intimate

"I wish we could have been more intimate. My husband was not too interested in being intimate with me."
                    -Julie, Environ. Compliance Inspector

Although touch was the number one topic mentioned by the women surveyed with regard to romance during pregnancy, men always mention intimacy. Dads-to-be or not, single or married, dating or celebrating their golden anniversaries, when it comes to romance, intimacy pops into the minds of men. And, that's due to the way men are wired. Sexual intimacy increases testosterone and dopamine levels in men, which leads to the release of endorphins in the brain.

But, when physical intimacy leads to a pregnancy, often, for both men and women, intimacy takes on new challenges. It's looked upon in a different light. It has more meaning. Your partner's breasts and vagina are no longer just recreational areas. They are looked at as functional.

Your intimate relationship will transform during pregnancy. Libidos may increase or decrease. Lubrication production will change. Your partner may become more, or less, orgasmic. You'll have to use creativity when it comes to positioning in the later months. Some men find all the changes alluring and sexy. Others look at the changes more as obstacles. Some even express fears over physical intimacy. Many pregnant women's ideas of intimacy will also fluctuate. Some have the insatiable libido of a bunny in heat. While others are experiencing nausea and awkwardness that keep the idea of romping between the sheets at bay. But one thing you can be sure of, be it sexual relations or merely a soft kiss, your pregnant partner desires intimacy, the need to have a close personal relationship with you, the father of her baby.

The Fear of Intercourse

"I could not get sex for anything. He was convinced that he would hurt the baby and poke her in the forehead."
-Jodi R., Homemaker

It makes sense. Doctors and midwives are asked it all the time. I haven't met a father yet who wasn't concerned: "If we have sex, can it hurt the baby?"

"There's no biological fact of that," says Jill Dozier, with nine years experience helping pregnant women as a doula, nurse, and certified midwife. "Baby can't get hurt during intercourse. Just let Mom call the shots."

The baby is comfortably cushioned in an amniotic fluid-filled sac within Mom's uterus. The uterus is sealed off from the outside world via a mucous plug. So, unless you're being excessively rough, there's no need to fear that you'll injure Mom or Baby during sexual intercourse. If you have a reason to be concerned, though, or if there are already any pregnancy complications, consult your ob-gyn before having sex.

Another concern dads experience with regard to sexual intercourse with their pregnant partners is the idea of Baby being "present." "Does the baby know we're having sex?" men ask. And the answer is a resounding, "No." Yet, although she doesn't know, for some men, it just doesn't feel right. They say it's like sneaking sex in the same room as their sleeping child.

If you want to be sexually intimate with your partner, you'll need to get past this obstacle. Baby has no idea that you're having sex. She has no concept of intercourse. And, even if she did, she'll have no memory of the act. The stigma lies within us. So, if we can get past it, we'll be making everyone happy. Men need the sexual release. According to midwife, Jill Dozier, Baby will enjoy the rocking motion. And, she may even enjoy the contractions during Mom's orgasm. Tracy Schmidt, who's had twenty-two years experience assisting over 1,500 couples as a natural childbirth educator assures that your pregnant partner can really use some intimate focus. And that "physical intimacy is really healthy for her."

"I almost had to beg him to make love to me sometimes, because he was afraid of hurting the baby. I found it very exciting to have sex without worrying about getting pregnant. I already was!"
-E. A., Marketing Associate

The Libido Factor

"During the first pregnancy I felt sexy the entire time, right up until delivery. My libido was a monster. He really didn't have to do anything. He could have just stood there in front of me. I was interested every single minute."
-Allison, Mother of Two

Wow! Every fella's dream, huh? I had no idea that a woman's libido was boosted during pregnancy, but there are many factors that contribute to this surge in sexual energy. Some are hormonal, others physiological, and yet others are mental. But, regardless of the reason, men need to know that many pregnant women have voracious sexual appetites, and if men are avoiding sex during this time, it can lead to self-esteem issues for Mom-to-be.

Some women will find that their sexual libido takes a nosedive during the first three months of pregnancy. The fatigue and vomiting, as well as breast tenderness contribute to the "I'm not in the mood" syndrome.

But, others will find that they are more sexual during that first trimester due to that same breast sensitivity, as well as hypersensitive vulva which have become engorged.

Most women, though, mentioned that it was indeed during that second trimester that their bodies truly kicked into sexual overdrive. Blood flow to a pregnant woman's sexual organs and breasts increase during the second trimester. Morning sickness has often subsided, estrogen and progesterone are still on the rise, and the couple is starting to feel a bit more at ease with the whole idea of the pregnancy.

Women often find sex pleasurable during pregnancy, sometimes more so than before they were pregnant, because of the vagina's increased lubrication production. Also, all of that extra blood flow helps some women become orgasmic for the first time. And, some, who've already had the pleasure of orgasm, may become multi-orgasmic.

A huge boost to the libido for both men and women is that the fear of becoming pregnant is gone. You can't get pregnant, because you already are. The concern about birth control has been eliminated. Spontaneity can take over. Once we experience less stress, we free our minds to enjoy more of what life has to offer, including sex.

Don't count out the fact that some women find the changes that they are going through wildly erotic. Knowing that she has created a life with you, may draw your partner closer to you emotionally, as well as sexually. The roundness of their bodies and fullness of their breasts sometimes allow pregnant women to feel more feminine, and, therefore, more sexy. Peter G., a Connecticut father of three, saw it in his wife, Fran, who loved being pregnant. She knew she was attractive: "She felt very sexy when she was pregnant."

"During pregnancy, I was so horny. And, it wasn't for just one part. It was the entire pregnancy, from beginning to end. I didn't have morning sickness, so sex was on my mind every time, ALL THE TIME. It was great sex, too. Not only did my husband get to be intimate with 'another body', I got to enjoy it without infidelity. It was a win-win for us both."
-Ana, Age 32

For Play

"A massage would make me feel like having sex."
-26 Year-Old "Mami"

Although your partner may have a voracious sexual appetite, even though she may be able to create lubrication like she's turning on a faucet, don't jump right in there with both feet. Pregnant women still want foreplay. Some will need it. Yet others still want to be held, caressed and massaged like "Mami".

Find out what it takes to relax your pregnant partner, to get her in the mood. Make the foreplay feel like it's for play, something fun. Some women will respond to light touches on their arms and neck. Others will become excited by their partners' kisses. Breast and genital stimulation work best for others. Oral sex is fine, but be sure not to blow into the vagina. This could force air to enter her blood stream and cause an embolism, which can be deadly to both Mom and Baby.

Just be sensitive to Mom-to-be. Rev up her engines a bit before you go for a drive. And, maybe Mom doesn't need to be warmed up. She may not have a cold engine. But, let her take the reigns. Just follow her lead, and you'll both enjoy intimate time together.

"He could have communicated clearly when he wanted to be intimate, whether or not he thought I was tired. I needed to know he was still attracted to me sexually."
-Jenna, Former Teacher

The Right Position

"He was aware of my increasing girth, and found ways to make our intimate times more enjoyable. We continued to be intimate right up to a few days before delivery. He found my pregnant body to be beautiful, sexy, and desirable and told me so everyday."
-Valerie, Property Manager

As you and your partner approach the late stages of pregnancy, you may find that if you're still having intercourse, the positions that used to do the trick, just don't seem to be right any longer. You two have become a pair of puzzle pieces that no longer fit together.

Don't let a bit of belly keep you from enjoying what could be some of your last intimate moments before Baby arrives. This is the time for creativity, ingenuity, and flexibility. It may also be the time to break out that sense of humor. Sex with your eight-month pregnant spouse can be very warm and loving, but also a challenge. Allow yourself to laugh and have fun during sex. It doesn't have to be serious. It's supposed to be enjoyable and make you feel good.

Try experimenting with different positions. Which ones will allow you both to feel pleasure while still feeling close? Remember, though, that pregnant women should avoid lying flat on their backs after the fourth month of pregnancy, during sex or anytime. The weight of the uterus puts pressure on major blood vessels.

Here are some tried and true pregnancy positions that you may want to start with. Have your partner on top while you lie on your back. This allows her to control the pace, and it frees your hands to rub her body and stimulate her breasts.

There's the rear entry position, which is very effective in late pregnancy. As your partner is on her hands and knees, you enter her from behind. With this position the belly really is no obstacle, but face-to-face contact is difficult.

Spooning is a branch of the "rear position" tree. You're still entering your partner from behind, so there's no cumbersome tummy to deal with, but when spooning, you are both lying on your sides. Because you don't need your hands or knees to keep you propped up, spooning can feel a bit more intimate to some couples. Hands are free to hug and stroke. There also seems to be a bit more body freedom.

Most importantly when finding new positions during pregnancy, make your partner feel sexually secure with herself and her body. Some women thrive on positions that flaunt their new bodies. Other women, like Deanna (next page) aren't so comfortable with their body transformations:

"My husband was aware of my insecurities about my changing body and would discreetly cover areas I was embarrassed by so that I could feel comfortable enough to be intimate."
-Deanna W., Age 35

When to Avoid Intercourse

"We had to refrain (from intercourse) due to premature contractions. So, I got a lot of awesome foot rubs and words of encouragement that it was gonna be o.k. And, it was."
-Cathy W., Stay At Home Mom

Although an extremely popular way to express intimacy, sexual relations may not always be pleasurable, possible, or advisable during pregnancy. The following are alternative ways to express intimacy with your pregnant partner. But, it's important to understand when and why sex may need to be avoided.

Refrain from intercourse:
• during the first trimester if you partner has experienced past miscarriages
• during the second and third trimesters, if she's carrying twins or her water breaks
• during her last trimester if she's had premature labor during past pregnancies

Be sure to consult with your wife's physician for your specific circumstance and any other kind of high-risk pregnancy.

Even during pregnancies that are not considered high risk, there are times when abstinence is advised. If your partner experiences vaginal bleeding or contractions, avoid vaginal penetration. Prostaglandin, a hormone present in semen, can cause her uterus to contract more, which can lead to early delivery.

Finally, there may be no medical reason for it, but you have to remember that each woman reacts differently to pregnancy. And, within each individual pregnancy, women react differently to the changes within the trimesters. So, she may experience awkwardness and discomfort. She may feel fatigued and nauseous. These do not lend themselves to an amorous evening.

Be understanding and flexible with your partner. Remember, sex changes during pregnancy. Expect the unexpected. As mentioned, listen to your partner. Read her body language. If sex isn't in the picture this night, this week, or even this month, don't take it personally. Show her your feelings, and romance her with alternative modes of intimacy.

"My husband was very loving during my pregnancy as we continued to have sex with less frequency, of course, but the romance was always there."

-A.C., General Manager

Alternative Modes of Intimacy

"I would have liked him to kiss me - anytime. We may not have been having a lot of physical intimacy late in pregnancy, but kisses and hugs help tell me that I'm loved."

-Lynne S., First Time Mom

As mentioned, there are circumstances when sexual intercourse is not medically recommended. And, pregnancy brings with it both physical and psychological conditions that make intercourse uncomfortable. Stretching pelvic ligaments, as well as when the baby's head is engaged in the pelvis, can make deep penetration unpleasant. Some women, and men for that matter, lose the desire for sexual intercourse due to anxiety over pregnancy and becoming new parents.

But, just because sexual intercourse is no longer an option doesn't mean intimacy needs to be out of the picture. If your partner is still sexually interested but penetration is not a choice, consider oral sex, if it's advisable, or even manual stimulation. If the sexual appetite has taken a sabbatical, there are other forms of non-sexual intimacy that will show your pregnant partner that she's being cared for and is special. Search for alternate ways of being intimate, close and romantic.

Many moms said that they craved hugs and kisses in lieu of physical intimacy. So, snuggle your partner's growing body. Touch her. You can also show your partner that, although you're unable to share the act of sex itself, that she's still sexy, as Tracy wished her husband had shown her:

"My husband could have bought me sexy and romantic nightwear that would have made me look and feel nice as I got larger."
-Tracy S., Leland, NC

10 Things You Need to Know About Intimacy During Pregnancy

1. Some studies show that couples who remain sexually active during pregnancy have lower rates of premature labor in comparison to those who abstain from sex.
2. You don't need birth control. Take advantage of this freedom.
3. Never underestimate the power of foreplay.
4. Let her be in charge of the pacing.
5. You won't hurt Baby as long as you're gentle.
6. Enjoy your partner's changing body.
7. Tell your partner how sexy she is.
8. Be careful with those sensitive nipples.
9. Baby has no idea of what you two are doing.
10. Be gentle, patient and keep a good sense of humor.

Your partner wants to be seen as more than a mom. She still wants to be seen as a woman!

5

Isn't She Lovely?

"My husband was always very encouraging, reminding me that my big tummy, my stretch marks, etc... were all indications of a beautiful process going on inside me, that any sign of this growth was gorgeous."

-Eliza L. R., California

Both times that my wife, Mary, was pregnant with our girls, I found her beautiful, radiant actually. And, I told her this, not because I wanted to build her self-confidence, but because it was true, because every time I looked at her, I couldn't help but stating the truth... she was absolutely lovely.

Therefore, Mary was never lacking positive comments regarding her outward appearance. That's why I was so stunned to learn how incredibly important those little comments are to a pregnant woman. Over one-third of the women surveyed either said that when their partners told them they were beautiful, they felt romanced, or that they weren't told it enough. So, even though you might think it, she wants you to tell her and show her that she's beautiful.

She Already Knows

"My husband would give me massages, bathe me, shave my legs in the shower for me since I could not reach, lay on the bed and 'talk' to the baby through my tummy, and he always commented on how beautiful I looked the bigger I got."

-T. S., Mother of Two Boys

Some pregnant women already know that they are beautiful. The fullness of their bodies as well as the knowledge that they are carrying a new life is the epitome of beauty in their eyes. Confidence and self-esteem levels skyrocket. They marvel at the changes in the mirror. They love putting on maternity clothes. They are beautiful, and they know it.

Allison of Portland, Maine not only felt beautiful, but she knew her pregnant body was sexy. So, if your partner is anything like Allison, does it mean you get a free ride on the "No Compliment" Ferry? Sorry, no seats available on that ride. You still need to let her know that you find her attractive. It's not enough that she thinks it herself. What about you, the father of her baby? Do you think she's pretty?

Allison's husband knew his wife found her pregnant body beautiful, but he would still tell her how marvelous she looked. No matter how high her level of self-esteem has reached, your pregnant partner is still fragile and being bombarded with an arsenal of hormones that could make anyone unstable. So, for the sake of romance, make it a point to tell her she's beautiful.

"He told me I was beautiful at least five times a day."
-Melissa B., 29 Year-Old Teacher

She Doesn't Know Yet

"My husband told me I looked young. It was romantic because when you become a mother, you suddenly enter a different role and feel much older and not as attractive."
-Nicole, Musician

Many women share Nicole's sentiments with regard to pregnancy and how they see themselves. This vision may not necessarily be the same sight the rest of the world sees, but with the added weight, the clumsiness, the morning sickness, the anxiety of becoming someone's mother and the sleepless nights, no matter how beautiful she may look to you, your partner may see a less attractive, aging woman on the other side of that mirror.

It's your job to convince her that not only is she still attractive, but also that pregnancy adds a new luster to her beauty.

Childbirth expert Tracy Schmidt adds that not only does telling your pregnant partner she's beautiful help her self-esteem, but it dispels the myth that her body is her enemy, which some women start to believe as pregnancy continues. "She'll feel more comfortable with her body if she believes it's attractive and healthy," says Schmidt, "and that will lead to a more positive birth experience. Besides, all of these wonderful comments are a good investment in your relationship. It builds trust and love that will continue even after Baby arrives."

The fourth month of pregnancy is the time for you to really kick the compliments into high gear. It's around this time that your partner will really begin to look pregnant. Although her hormone levels may subside, she may still feel emotional and vulnerable for the duration of her pregnancy. So, make an effort to point out how your pregnant partner's beauty shines.

"More hugs and more compliments."
-J.C., Age 28

Simple: Just Say It

"I wish he'd taken the time to tell me I was beautiful. Pregnancy is so weird to your body. It is difficult to feel attractive, especially in the last trimester."
-R. H., Age 31

So, tell her. Tell her. Tell her. Let her know she's beautiful. She wants to know you find her attractive. As you know, many pregnant women are self-conscious of the physical changes that are taking place. They are very aware of their changing bodies, and they're being pumped with enough hormones to keep a small poultry farm in business.

Your partner's emotional and psychological well-being are crucial for both her and the baby during these nine months. A little "you've got this attractive glow about you" and a simple "I can't remember a time you looked more radiant" can work wonders for your partner's psyche. And, it doesn't take much effort or time on your part. Heartfelt compliments like these boost your partner's serotonin levels. When serotonin levels rise, stress levels fall. She becomes optimistic, content, and comforted. Telling your partner that you find her attractive can be one of the simplest and most powerful ways of bringing romance to this and future pregnancies.

Pregnant women not only want to hear that they are beautiful, but they need to hear it often. With so many changes and stages that take place through pregnancy, you can't assume that a compliment you gave her last week still packs the same wallop it did when you said it. "Sure," she thinks, "I was attractive then, but I've gained two more pounds and have a new varicose vein. Does he *still* find me attractive?"

Tell her often, and, to make things interesting, mix up your approaches. Sure, she'll appreciate a "you sure are pretty" everyday, but the impact will be even stronger if she hears it one day as she leaves for work and the next day when she opens her sack lunch to find a quick "You are my beautiful wife" scribbled on her napkin.

Send her an email telling her how you've grown more attracted to her during pregnancy. Or, call her from work just to tell her you can't wait to see her gorgeous face and rub her sexy tummy later that night. Write her a poem about her beauty, or, better yet, write her a letter and mail it to your home.

Kiss your partner before you go to sleep, and tell her she's beautiful. When you see her full body stepping nude from the shower tell her she's beautiful. When she wakes up in the morning with her mussed up hair and no make-up, tell her she's beautiful

Tell her. Tell her. Tell her. Because she *is* beautiful!

"He told me at least twice a day how beautiful I was and that he was attracted to my changing body."
                                                    -J.H., Full Time Mom

Actions Can Speak Volumes

"He wanted to take lots of pictures of me and my pregnant belly. He eventually put these pictures into a little photo album. I found this to be romantic because it showed that he appreciated my new body."
                                        -M. L., Elementary School Teacher

As well as telling your partner how beautiful she is, sometimes your actions will let her know that you not only appreciate her new body, but that you also find it attractive.

Many dads-to-be will ask their partners to expose their swelling tummies to capture on film. The roundness and fullness are compelling enough to display in an album or in a frame. Be it a tasteful black and white shot of the beauty of pregnancy or a weekly chronicle of her growing mid-section, Mom-to-be will feel delighted and flattered to be asked to be the model for your photos. You feel her body should be the central focus of an image that captures a single moment in time. Although you're not saying it in words, she will feel attractive and beautiful.

Along the same lines, there are companies now that will capture your wife's torso via plaster molds. Let's say you suggest a plaster mold of Mom-to-be's growing mid-section, so you can have a memory of this miraculous time. How will she feel? You love her body and its changes so much that you want a life-size cast of it for all time. This shows her that you find her attractive and beautiful.

Many women I've spoken to mention that their husbands or boyfriends stopped buying them cute outfits once they became pregnant. This makes pregnant Mom feel as though her man doesn't find her worthy enough to wear attractive clothing. Therefore, she no longer feels pretty.

Buy her a cute outfit. Pregnant women still want sexy lingerie. Just because she's gained 35 pounds, she's not condemned to wear a muumuu. Find something that will show some skin. Let her bare her shoulders. Find a skirt to show off her legs. Some pregnant women love to wear form-fitting, slinky dresses out on the town, showing off their new bulge. A great place to start is Mimi Maternity (MimiMaternity.com or call 1-877-646-4666).

When you buy her a cute outfit, you're telling your pregnant partner that she is cute, that you still find her attractive, that she doesn't have to wait nine months to be beautiful again. She's beautiful now!

Finally, I'd like to mention it again. You will tell her she's beautiful again and again, the more you touch your pregnant wife at home and in public. We don't touch people or things we find repulsive or ugly. Yet, the more attractive something is, the closer to it we wish to be, and the more we touch it. So, through touch, let the mother-to-be of your baby know she's the most beautiful thing to walk this earth.

"When I was pregnant, one of the nicest things my husband did for me that made me feel sexy and desirable was when he polished my toenails for me (which I couldn't reach anymore!), and then he gave me a wonderful foot massage, commenting the entire time how sexy my feet were. Not only did the attention to my feet feel wonderful, his eagerness to pay attention to me made me feel attractive."
-L. S., Mom For Eleven Months

Find Beauty In The Process

"He talks a lot about how amazing my body is doing the job of pregnancy."
-Thalia, Mom-To-Be

There are those of you who look at a pregnant woman and can't help but smile. Be it your partner or not, you find a woman with child a beautiful sight.

Then, there are those of you who don't see the beauty. You see a big woman with swollen ankles. You see a waddle instead of a swish. You see a woman with varicose veins and odd food cravings. You aren't evil. You can't force a person to see the beauty in a flower. You can't make a person love the flavor of rocky road ice cream. Therefore, you can't blame a man for not seeing the physical beauty of a pregnant woman.

But, you can blame him for not seeing the inner beauty of his pregnant partner. Remember, no matter how her body changes, how her moods may swing, how anxious she may become, she is the same woman you decided to have a baby with. And, you probably chose her not only for her physical beauty, but also for her inner beauty.

The woman you fell in love with is still in there. Behind that growing uterus and amidst the onslaught of hormones, your beautiful partner is waiting for you. Pregnancy will change a lot, but it won't change either one of you as people. Your cores will remain the same. You'll be the same man she loves, and she'll be the same beautiful woman you fell in love with.

If you are one of those men who have difficulty finding her outer beauty, look at her physical changes in a new light. Notice the symmetry in her body and how nature has created a perfect vessel for your baby. Enjoy her taut roundness, and notice how the curves flow into each other. Think about the fact that one of millions of your sperm found her one egg at just the right time. And, those two reproductive cells have formed to create a brand new human life, with hair and fingers and a personality, your baby. Look at her and see the beauty that is the miracle of life. When you look at your pregnant partner with all of the changes, see her body as the receptacle that not only keeps Baby safe, but that holds Baby as she percolates to the perfect brew. There is beauty in pregnancy.

"He says that I look the most beautiful he's ever seen me when I'm pregnant. He loves the fact that I'm carrying his unborn child and thinks it makes me gorgeous."

-Pamela, 36 Year-Old Scientist

Just Can't Weight

"I wish he would have not spoken so much about my weight gain during the entire pregnancy. It's only natural that your body will change and things expand."

-Christina, 21 Year-Old Receptionist

Christina is absolutely right. It's only natural. That's what her body needs to do during pregnancy. Your partner is suppose to gain weight, not just the weight of her unborn baby, but she may retain water. Her breasts will become larger. Weight is gained as the placenta and uterus grow. She'll also be adding 40 to 50 percent more blood to her total blood volume.

Although it's 100% natural and your partner knows it, she may still feel self-conscious about the weight gain. These new sizes in clothing may be foreign to her. And, although her head is telling her it's natural, her heart may be a bit uneasy about the changes.

Your job is not to point out the weight gain making her feel more critical of herself, but instead to point out her changes in a flattering manner. You don't have to pretend not to notice the weight gain. Just don't look at it in a negative light. Try the "glass half-full" approach. Instead of, "God, your stomach is really getting fat," try, "I love touching your round tummy."

There are occasions when a pregnant woman gains more weight than is necessary, or even healthy, for her and the baby. If this is a concern, instead of going straight to Mom-to-be, check out some pregnancy books first. See what they have to say. Weight gain fluctuates drastically from woman to woman.

You can also check out pregnancy sites on-line (like AmericanBaby.com, BabyCenter.com, and BabyZone.com) or even call your wife's ob-gyn, mid-wife, doula, or childbirth coach. If your research leads you to believe her weight gain is unhealthy, there are two trains of thought on how to handle this. Based upon my experience and speaking with moms and new moms, I say to bring up your concern with her ob-gyn so *the doctor* can broach the subject with your partner. That way it's coming from a professional. It's not personal; it's medical. Besides, you're going to have to go home with this woman. What man wants to go to sleep in a house with a pregnant woman he's told was too fat? You'd have to sleep with one eye open!

But, if you don't like the idea of talking to the doctor without your partner's knowledge, you might want to broach the subject in a straightforward and loving way: "Honey, you know that I think you're the most beautiful woman in the world, but I'm concerned about... What do you think?" If this elicits a negative response, *then* you might consider consulting with her ob-gyn.

No matter your approach, remember, during pregnancy (and when she's not pregnant, for that matter) what you do in your relationship should be done out of love, not to hurt, cause pain or ridicule.

"My husband made me feel comfortable with my changing body using one simple technique; every time I said I felt 'big' or 'fat', he replied very gently, 'No, honey, you are <u>pregnant</u>!' It sounds like such a small thing, but it made a world of difference in how I saw myself and how I believed he saw me."

-Caroline A., 34 Year-Old Manager

9 Ways To Tell Her She's Beautiful

1. Show her off. Take her out and introduce her as your beautiful wife.

2. Buy her cute outfits and sexy undies.
3. Say these words: "You are beautiful".
4. Touch her often.
5. Let her know you love her changing body.
6. Kiss the woman, for goodness sake!
7. Tell her that she's got a glow about her.
8. Take her picture often.
9. Pay attention to her.

"Tell me I look beautiful. In late pregnancy I felt puffy and swollen - not attractive. Having my husband still want to touch me would make me feel desirable and loved."

-Lynne, 35 Year-Old First-Time-Mom

6

She Can Count On You

"I had heard horror stories of friends who went through their pregnancies virtually alone, with little support from their spouses. My husband knew I was nervous, even before conception, and promised me he would always be there, and we would handle any question together. To this day, he has been true to his word. For me, that is one of the most romantic gifts he could have given me, his promise to be a father involved."

-V. S., Age 46

What women have told me they mean when they say they want to count on their men is the comfort of having someone in their corner, a partner that they can rely on, through the easy days as well as the tough ones.

When a man can do this for his partner, she feels protected and is having her needs met, which is a serotonin enhancer. And, when your pregnant partner's serotonin levels rise, she's less anxious and more positive. An added benefit for men is that when we act as the pillars of strength in our relationships (the Superman to her Lois Lane) we feel as though we're serving and protecting our partners. This increases our testosterone levels, which allows us to become more caring and compassionate. Endorphins are released; we feel terrific, and romance stays alive.

Sometimes your partner will need your encouragement or a kind word. She'll want you to participate in the pregnancy and offer her the support she'll need. There will be times that she may doubt herself and will rely on you to pick her back up afterward. Sometimes you'll need to be her Man of Steel, while other times she'll require an ear for listening, more of a Clark Kent-type.

You must be her stability, the pillar of strength and support these nine months. Show her through your actions that you are here for her and the baby, and it will build her confidence that she has chosen the right man as the father of her child.

Availability

"Whether he was afraid, overwhelmed, or immature (my spouse) actually distanced himself (during my pregnancy). Since I went from thin and active to gaining weight and exhausted, he didn't embrace the changes or find them a miracle, like I did"
-Susan, Age 40 from California

Susan's husband distanced himself from his wife during her pregnancy. She told this to me ten years later. She hadn't forgotten. Your partner not only wants you to avoid distancing yourself from her, but she wants you to become closer. Become available to her.

Pregnancy can be an unsteady time, and your wife will want to know that there will be someone around for her, preferably you. If you can, avoid staying late at work or going in on weekends. Minimize nights out with the boys. And, when you can't be there for her, call. Call her during a break at work. If you're stuck in traffic dial her number on the cell. Knowing that you're thinking of her and being able to communicate with her even by phone when necessary, will give your pregnant partner the comfort of knowing you are available for her.

Maybe your partner doesn't say so, but she needs you. Of course she could make it through this pregnancy without your support. Women experience pregnancy alone all the time and survive it. But, she needs your emotional support for her romantic sanity. And, you being around, putting out the effort of physically and emotionally being there for her, you are giving her that support.

"He attended marriage and family counseling weekly until the month before birth."
-Jenna H., Mom for Six Months

Communication

"He was a good listener and tender when I was moody and hormonal."

-J. H., Age 27

Pregnant or not, women want men who will express their feelings and who are astute listeners. Saying, "I'm listening", while you watch the game, or responding with monosyllabic answers does not make a strong communicator. In any relationship, but especially during pregnancy, men need to be attentive and truly hear what their partners are trying to express to them. Turn off the T.V. Look her in the eyes, and listen. Nod your head so she knows you're still with her. You can also reach out and touch her if it feels right. But, be sure you are hearing what she's saying. Childbirth expert Tracy Schmidt advises, "Dads-to-be need to be attentive when she talks about her changing body, fears, excitement, etc..."

Now, the biggest mistake we men often make after "listening", especially if what we heard we perceive as problematic, is trying to fix it. We can't help it. It's our testosterone kicking in. If we solve the problem, we feel useful and helpful and our brain rewards us with endorphins. Someone tells us a problem, so we assume they want us to solve it. Not always the case! Sometimes women tell us "what's wrong" as a way to help them deal with it themselves. They want us to be sympathetic to their plight and not always be the duct tape to life's mishaps. So, unless she says these words, "What should I do?" refrain from fixing her problem.

"Then, what do I do instead?" you ask. Rephrase the problem so she knows you're listening. Ask questions about it. Let her come to her own resolution should she choose so. If not, be there for her as her security blanket, her walking diary, someone she can open up to without feeling scared, defensive, or embarrassed.

The flip side to listening is expressing your own feelings about the pregnancy to your partner. Men tend to "bottle up", while women tend to "pour out". When we bottle up, women are wondering what we're thinking, how we're feeling. If you're a man who's had trouble opening up in the past, this is the time to step out of your comfort zone. Invariably, you must be experiencing strong feelings about being a dad: anxiety, excitement, fear, relief. She wants to know. Yes, even the anxiety, and fear. When you open up to her and tenderly speak your heart, even if the topic isn't all nurseries and baby names, Mom-to-be knows you're part of this pregnancy, that you're not just passing it all off onto her, and that you've been thinking about it, too.

Psychologist, Dr. Juan R. Riker, advises that this might be easier said than done. "Some men may be aware that they have some, or all, of these feelings, but have no idea how to express them, or may even feel completely numb and are unaware that these feelings exist." So, the first step is identifying the feelings. Then, try to articulate them to your partner.

When Mom-to-be knows what's on your mind, she can share her feelings, too. Feelings are out in the open, everything's on the table, trust and honesty are apparent. And, suddenly, you grow even closer as a couple, and that, my friend, is of utmost importance. Although during pregnancy the focus is on pregnant Mom and the new baby, the most important relationship is the one between you and your partner. A strong and loving relationship between Mom and Dad keeps the bonds of family from becoming brittle. It teaches Baby how to love. And, it brings Mom and Dad closer as a twosome.

So, share your thoughts and dreams. Let Mom know that she and Baby are on your mind. Valerie S. can recall the openness between her and her husband during her pregnancy fourteen years prior: "He would get teary knowing that I was carrying the child that we had made together in love and would share that with me."

Open up to Mom-to-be. Ask her how she's feeling. Then, truly listen to her response. When she asks you questions, don't skirt the issue, shy away, or answer abruptly. Communicate with her. She'll find it romantic.

"My husband is not very verbal, but I think more intimate talks about my feelings and fears about the pregnancy would really have added to the romance."

-A. Cedeno, Age 38

In Courage

"I would have loved dinner out and candles (even though he's not too keen on them), or just a card or words of encouragement on paper."

-C. W., Age 40

When you encourage someone you're almost speaking to their heart in the language of "Courage." You give them confidence and strength. And, the heart understands because when you encourage you're speaking "In Courage".

Encouragement is the uncle of communication, but this is the uncle you always look forward to seeing at the annual family picnic. He's the one who makes you feel great about yourself, never a hurtful or mean thing to say. And, when you leave, you feel inspired and powerful. He's the uncle who makes you feel that you can do anything you set your mind to.

We all need uncles like this. But, a pregnant woman often needs encouragement even more so than the average Joan Public. Encourage her in any aspect that she may doubt her abilities or feel she can't perform or complete. If the two of you smoked or drank before pregnancy, assure her that you know she can abstain. And, show her that you can, too.

If she's fearful about the delivery process, encourage your partner by telling her that she is strong, that she can do this, that women less motivated and less determined than she have done it. Let her know that her body was made for this process.

If she's having excess stress, she'll appreciate your encouragement like 36-year-old student, Sabina, did when she just couldn't seem to chill out. "(My husband) encouraged me to go to the gym and to relax." Just a little push, some encouragement, can make any of us, but most of all our pregnant partners, get over that hump of doubt and down the positive slope.

Your pregnant partner may need you to remind her of who she is. You probably know her better than anyone else. Draw on all you know of her. Remind her how she's been able to handle stress in the past. Tell her how great she's doing. When she's practicing her breathing, encourage her. When she is eating right, encourage her. When she feels she wants to take that much needed nap, encourage her.

As dads-to-be, we may not all speak the same language, but we can all speak to the future moms of our babies in ways that will encourage them. Speak to your partner gently. Speak to her in love. Speak to her "in Courage".

"I had been an only child and was not used to small children. (My husband) made me feel confident and unafraid during my pregnancy that I would handle childbirth, and we would stumble together learning how to raise a child."
-Val, Mom For Fourteen Years

Compliments

"Positive affirmations - I felt so sick throughout my pregnancy, that any kind words and gestures of understanding would have made a difference."
-Martha L. S., Pilates Instructor

If encouragement is the positive uncle in the family of communication, compliments are the grandmas of the clan. You loved being with Grandma because she always made you feel warm and cared for. She raved about your haircut and the clothes you wore. She was proud of you for getting that first base hit in little league and for getting a job that paid over minimum wage.

Grandmas compliment. They see whatever it is you're interested in and make you feel good about it. We all need grandmas that make us feel this way. But, if your partner's grandma isn't around (or even if she is, for that matter), it's your job to shower her with compliments. Then, dry her with the towels of self-confidence.

Women tell me that when their men notice even the smallest accomplishments or comment on even the slightest effort, it makes them feel cared for and loved. It keeps them going through the difficult weeks, and it inspires them to reach the end.

As previously mentioned, compliment her on her beauty inside and out. Tell her you're proud of how she's stayed clear of cigarettes. Let her know you've noticed how she's eating healthy for her and the baby. Leave her a note telling her that she's doing great making it to her weekly pregnancy aerobics class. But, above all, compliment her on her strength. Tell her that you're amazed at how well she's dealing with the stress, her changing body and the lack of sleep.

Even if she's having difficulty with these areas, compliment her anyway. Often, when we know someone else thinks we're doing well (even when we don't think we are, ourselves) we step into that role that the other person sees. Words of encouragement can become self-fulfilling prophecies: "Oh, he thinks I'm handling the stress well? I guess maybe I am." Suddenly, she sees herself as a stress-handler, and the next time stress knocks at her door, she tells it, "No one's home." She *becomes* a stress-handler.

Compliment her when she's doing well. Compliment her when she's struggling. Compliments make us feel good. Grandma knows best.

"He told me how strong I was. I felt like we were falling in love for the second time."

-S. E., Teacher

Share The Experience

"He attended <u>every</u> appointment and birth class to show support for me and the baby."
                                        -Jen, Stay-at-Home Mom

A lot of men have told me, "If I could be the pregnant one, I would." The women I've spoken with have responded, "That's hogwash! He knows he'll never get pregnant, so it's an easy comment to make." Looks like we'll never truly know if men would take over the payments if Mom could switch the pregnancy mortgage over to his name.

But there are ways to get as involved as possible. This will make Mom feel as though she's not riding this elevator alone, because that's the last thing we want for our pregnant spouses. Although we can't carry Baby, we're just as responsible for the pregnancy as Mom is. We need to step up and do our part, not just for the sake of romance, but because it's our responsibility; it's our partner, and it's our baby.

The best way to share in your partner's experience is by getting involved as much as possible. Learn what's going on inside of her. A terrific NOVA video every dad-to-be should view, called *The Miracle of Life*, takes you through a sixty minute journey starting with sperm and egg introductions, right to the birth of the baby. It's available on many sites online, including Amazon.com.

Alison Stiles, part-time waitress and bartender, had a husband who was very involved: "He read all the same books I did and then tried to learn more, come back and show me what he knew." Read up on the baby, how big she is, what parts are developing, what she's doing in there.

Do whatever it takes to make it to the doctor visits. At the beginning of pregnancy, many men make time to get off work or to sneak away to accompany Mom to her appointments. But after the ultrasound appointments and a few waiting rooms of women with swollen ankles, the novelty can wear thin, and suddenly ob-gyn visits are no longer a priority for Dad-to-be.

Granted, sometimes it truly is nearly impossible to attend the appointments, especially when they're only a week apart at the end of pregnancy, but try to manipulate your schedule to make it possible to join Mom. Let your spouse know this is a priority for you so she can try to make appointments that will fit your schedule. You may have to miss one or two prenatal appointments, but don't skip out on the one when you first hear your baby's heartbeat (around the twelfth week) or when you can see baby (the twentieth week). These are moments in your life you can't afford to miss!

When Mom attends childbirth class, be there with her. These classes not only teach her how to breathe and relax, but they also teach her coach how to help her through delivery. Being your partner's birthing coach will raise your relationship to a new level. She's not delivering this baby alone. She needs you there to help her, to remind her, to relax her. The coach is a crucial member of the delivery team. Go to the childbirth classes. Then, at home, practice what you've learned. You will be showing Mom-to-be not only that you will support her during delivery, but that you are sharing her experience now.

Finally, Mom will probably start nesting late in pregnancy: tidying up, getting the nursery in order, buying diapers and wipes at the last minute. Don't leave her to nest alone. Share it with her. If she wants Baby's room green instead of yellow, get out the brushes and start painting. If she's heading off to Babies 'R Us, drive her and be sure you pick out at least one outfit. When you see a toy or stuffed animal you think would be a charming addition to Baby's already growing collection, bring it home. Part of the pregnancy experience is the focus on Baby. So focus on him.

I used to think that it would only be fair to have one parent experience pregnancy (nine months of nausea, edema, anxiety, clumsiness, back pain, sleeplessness, etc...) while the other experienced delivery (four to 36 hours of intense pressure and discomfort, being stretched in ways that would baffle Silly Putty). But since Nature has its own ways of doing things, which seem to have been working for quite some time, I decided that a visit to the ob-gyn, reading up on pregnancy, and purchasing a layette comes in at a close second.

"My second pregnancy was not planned. My husband, being as 'Type A' as you can get, had a very difficult time coming to terms with this 'surprise'. He wrote me a poem about two weeks after we found out I was pregnant that brought tears to my eyes and made me feel so close to him. The poem was about how he was ready mentally, physically, and emotionally to be a dad all over again. I found this romantic because that's when I knew we would experience 'round two' together."

-Maria P., Age 35

Don't Forget Baby

"He sang a song that he made up: 'We're Having a Little Baby'. It always made me laugh. I felt like we were falling in love for the second time."

-S. E., Age 32

One out of every five women surveyed found that when her man either shopped for, or talked to, the bundle of joy through Mama's tummy, it was romantic. And, that's because when we show that we care about Baby, we're showing Mom that we'll be caring fathers. A caring father adds stability to a pregnant woman's unstable world. By focusing on the baby you've never met, you're showing love for a being based solely on the fact that you created it with her. You love Baby, so you must love Mom.

When you focus on your unborn child, you can't help but focus on the vessel housing him, your partner. There are simple, nurturing, and effective ways to focus on Baby. Already mentioned is talking to Baby through Mom's tummy. Make it a ritual. Tell Baby about your day. Rub Mama's tummy as you speak so not only Baby can associate your voice to the touch, but also to soothe Mom with the caress.

Some dads-to-be will start a nightly ritual of reading a bedtime story to Baby or will sing to their offspring. Personally, I enjoyed counting to my girls. I would feel Mom's tummy for a bulge, and I'd gently press as I counted to five. Then, my wife and I would wait anxiously for a response. Would she "count" back? If there were a kick or two, I'd count them aloud to the bulge in the tummy. Mom and I would be delighted imagining our geniuses en-utero.

Some say the singing, reading, and counting help to build an early learning foundation. Others say the baby's too young to benefit from it all. But, what it definitely does is gives Baby a chance to become acclimated to Dad's voice. There's usually a lot of touching, so there's a bonding effect between Mom and Dad. And, also, Mom can feel a warmth knowing her man and her baby are building a bond.

Look through name books with Mom. Be part of the naming process. Go through your family's names. Go through her family's names. Look at the meanings and histories of names in one of the many "Baby Names" books you can pick up at your local bookstore.

To keep your relationship strong and romantic do not cause the naming of Baby to become a struggle; you fight for one name and she fights for another. On the other hand, don't leave it all up to her, either. Find a happy place in the middle where you both have a say in the name, and compromise, if you must. You don't want either of you to resent hearing this name the rest of your lives.

When you focus on Baby even before her arrival, Mom sees that you're already a dad involved. A man with a cape... Super Dad.

"Things that my husband could have done to be more romantic would just be to spend more time with me, talking to my belly, and rubbing my feet."

-Paula C., Office Manager

9 Ways To Let Mom Know She Can Count On You

1. Tell her your inner feelings about the pregnancy and becoming a dad.
2. Call a local radio station and dedicate a song to her expressing how you feel about her (e.g. "The Wind Beneath My Wings").
3. Attend childbirth classes with her.
4. Listen with your heart, and don't feel compelled to "fix" things.
5. Make her a tape or CD with songs that will make her feel good about herself, her pregnancy and your relationship.
6. Write a poem about her strengths and get it put into a candle (CandleLightMessages.com).
7. Read books on pregnancy and the developing fetus/embryo.
8. Take out a newspaper ad about how awesome your wife has been through pregnancy. Then, be sure she sees it.
9. Buy a bunch of inspirational cards and stash them away. When your partner is feeling discouraged or moody, write something to perk her up, and leave the card where you know she'll find it.

"Understand that (pregnancy) is an emotional roller coaster, and we need support, and lots of cuddles and kisses."
-Rebecca H., Mom For Six Months

7

It's About Time

"I would have liked it had he planned a day trip for us to be together, telling me that he wants to spend some quality couple time alone before the baby arrives. This would be romantic because it would show me that he still values me for me, not just as the mother of his unborn child."

-Lynne S., Associate Director

The following applies to all parents-to-be, but especially to first time moms and dads: spend as much romantic time together as you can before Baby arrives. You may envision idyllic evenings as the three of you snuggle together on the couch, each reading your own book and enjoying the company of the other two. You may dream of leaving the baby with the sitter as the two of you spend a night out together focused solely on each other. You may plan on returning to your intimate times in the evening while your child sleeps serenely in his crib beneath glowing ceiling stars and a mobile that matches the wall borders.

And, in a perfect world, you and your spouse will be able to enjoy time together, but in the world where most of us raise our children, no books get read on that couch but Baby's, if you're lucky. And, although you may work up enough nerve to leave Baby with a sitter as you dash out to dinner, the dining conversation may be more on the lines of, "How do you think he's doing?" and "Do you think we should call and check on him?".

By the way, do not count on, never rely on, intimacy when Baby sleeps. Somehow, I'm not sure if it's some kind of messaging Mom inadvertently sends through the breast milk, or if Baby is just reacting to Dad's excitement realizing he's moments away from a romp in the haystack, but Baby knows when you plan to have sex when she sleeps. So, plan all you want. Check on her sixteen times if you wish to be sure she's really out. Tip toe, whisper, and keep the noise to a minimum as much as you like. The moment things begin to heat up, the instant you forget Baby's in the other room, the second you let yourself go and focus solely on your partner, that's Baby's cue, screaming from the top of her lungs, pulling the emergency brake on the railroad car of passion.

The point? Get it in now, before Baby arrives. Spend time together, not just as parents-to-be, but as the couple you first were. I don't mean to frighten you. The other day, a friend of my wife and mine described it so well: "When it was just the two of us it was wonderful. After we had Amanda, it was a different kind of wonderful."

You will get your "couple time" back someday, but it may be quite some time. You will cherish life as parents when Baby arrives, but until then, cherish your one-on-one time with your pregnant partner.

Get Away

"(My husband) took me to a health spa for a week, and I had lots of massages, swimming, lovely meals, and was pampered to death. He doesn't really like that sort of thing, so he just waited around for me. It just made me realize how much he loved me... We had a fabulous room and a fabulous time."
-R. H., Age 31 From England

What better way to escape the confines that life bestows upon us than with a getaway? Pregnant or not, we tend to place our relationships and romance far down on our priority lists, thinking, "We'll get to it soon," but often never getting to it at all because of work, bills, errands, television programs, walking the dog, household chores, and being pregnant. I mean there are the nursery, the name choosing, the childbirth classes, the showers, and the Thank You cards that need to be written. There's rarely time to focus on that other adult in the house, the one who helped create this new life that everyone's fussing over.

"We feared losing our one-on-one time a bit with our first (child)," explains father of three, Peter Greenberg of Connecticut, "but we squeezed in a bunch of vacations before each baby was born." And, what about the kids? They just dropped them off at the grandparents'.

A trip allows us to reconnect as a couple and releases us from the confines of daily responsibilities: no dinners to cook or house to clean, no phone calls to make or mail to read, no laundry to wash and no work to bring home. All that's left is all that there was at the beginning of your relationship: just the two of you. When we release ourselves from the stresses of life, we allow romance to once again become a priority in our lives.

When you decide to sweep her away, you'll bring new life to your relationship. You'll fall in love all over again. And, she'll appreciate being treated like the woman you met so long ago.

Now, your trip doesn't have to be a three-week excursion to twelve European nations. And, you don't have to take her on a fourteen-day Alaskan cruise. What truly matters is that the two of you are getting away, together, without life interrupting the romance that's been itching to be scratched.

If you've got the time and money, go big. But, do refrain from traveling too far from your home after the 35th week, in case your partner experiences early labor. You need to be close to your hospital and to her doctor.

But, if you can only pull off a weekend trip, an overnight stay at a local Bed and Breakfast, or a trip to a day spa, remember it's not so much about how long you're gone, but more about your focus. Give her your presence and make it easy for her to offer you hers. Forget about the rest of the world. Rediscover the woman you fell in love with and let her find that man who swept her off her feet.

Upon your return to reality, you'll probably end up in the same old grind: work, chores, and crib building. But, when you look at her, and your eyes meet as you pass each other at the refrigerator (she on her way to answer the phone, you heading out the door to wash the car), you'll both know why you're in this together. You'll see not just the woman you share the house with, but also the woman you chose as the mother of your baby. And, you'll smile, appreciating the time you had during your getaway.

"He planned a special, last weekend together for us at a resort in Palm Springs."

-Jenna, 27 Year-Old Former Teacher

Date Her

"He takes me out on dates so that we have as much time together as we can before the baby gets here."

-Sylvia, Chemist

Take her out before Baby arrives. Remember when you were courting? You'd take her to dinner, a concert, maybe a movie. Pregnant women enjoy food, music, and film just as much as any other woman. The difference: soon her focus will predominantly be aimed at the new life you two will have created.

Besides, this is not just a countdown of your last days alone. The women I speak with say that they *want* that special time with their men. They love having their partners take them out and show them off, in essence saying, "Look world, this is my beautiful, pregnant wife, and I'm the luckiest man in the universe!"

Although it's not a getaway, trip, or vacation, a date also allows Mom-to-be to forget about the regular stresses of everyday. Someone else cooks and cleans the dishes. There's no phone to answer and no anxiety over the baby. There's just one-on-one time with the man she loves.

So, find out what she wants to do. Ask her on a date. Put it on the calendar or in your planner. If you've got other kids, get a baby-sitter or drop them off at Grandma's. Get all gussied up. Shave. Pull out that old bottle of cologne. Make her feel special. Then, enjoy her company. Don't just be next to her; be *with* her. Be present, and enjoy the time you have on this date with the woman you love.

"Taking me out to a fancy dinner would have been romantic. I still want to be the sexy girl he met and fell in love with, even if I am about to be a 'mom'."

-L. S., Age 35

Get Out

"He took me for long walks on the beach."

-Sabina, Mom-To-Be

Time spent with your pregnant partner doesn't have to be extravagant or fancy. It doesn't have to cost much or even anything at all. When women speak to me about spending time with their men, it's about quality, no distractions or diversions. It's time meant to share thoughts and feelings, to add layers to the bond built between them and their men. It's to share a story about their day or to hear their partner tell a joke. The time is meant for holding hands and touching.

Some of the best ways to share these private moments is just by getting out. Moms, moms-to-be, and new moms tell me time and again how important their nightly walks with their husbands are. Not only are they healthy, helping Mom to keep fit while burning calories and allowing her blood to circulate, which minimizes the likelihood of edema, but they are also time away from phones, TV's, bills, work, chores, and children.

So, walk when and where you can. If she'll enjoy the crispness of dawn, go for an early morning walk. Maybe she's more into sunsets, so walk at dusk. Walk in a park or maybe down along the beach. The setting and time alone can add a lot to the romantic nature of the walk.

But, you know, getting out doesn't even really have to be about the walk. Take a blanket and watch the waves from a cliff. Or, lay back in chaise lounge chairs on the back lawn and count shooting stars. Drive to the highest point in town and watch the sunset from the front seat of your car as you listen to the Oldies station.

Find a spot that works for the two of you. Go when it's the ideal time. Turn off the cell phone and be together. Good chance she'll not only feel the buds of romance blossoming, but you may, too.

"We went for walks and he would go my pace instead of walking his usual pace."
                                        -Jen H., California

"Fit" It In

"Pool-time together - We'd swim together or he'd gently push me around the pool on a floaty."
                        -Jenna, 27 Year-Old Former Teacher

As mentioned, walking is a terrific way for pregnant Mom to stay fit while spending quality one-on-one time with Dad. Exercise is crucial for a pregnant woman, but it has to be geared specifically to her and her condition. Although Mom may feel, now that she holds the seed of life germinating within her, that she can accomplish anything, in reality her body heats up faster, and the muscles may fatigue quicker. Since her ligaments are being pulled and stretched, she may feel a bit more tender. Her fitness regimen may need to be altered to low impact activities that will still keep the blood pumping, keeping her body, and the baby's, strong and healthy.

There are exercise books as well as videos and classes designed exclusively for the prenatal mom. Although your partner may benefit from them, there's one thing they lack... you.

If you are able to join your spouse as she works to keep healthy, you are not only showing her love, but you're keeping her company and spending quality time with her before Baby arrives.

Most men aren't quite comfortable joining their spouses at the local YMCA's aerobics class filled with pregnant women and their protruding bellies. Many men won't even join their spouses in doing leg lifts and side stretches if the video shows spandex or the book mentions the word "uterus".

But, there are other ways to show romance and spend time with your partner as you both keep fit, while still maintaining your masculinity.

The swimming pool is a great way to stay fit for both men and women, parents-to-be or not. It's especially beneficial to pregnant Mom. Swimming is an activity in which you use almost all of your body. It's low-impact. And pregnant women love the buoyancy. Suddenly, all that extra weight is lifted and she has some of the physical freedom again that has slowly been slipping away. One word of caution, though: don't offer Mom a smoothie, or any drink for that matter, before the swim. Mom's got enough pressure on her bladder as it is, but when we get into the pool, the water puts pressure on our bodily fluids, which need an escape, usually through the bladder.

As mentioned, walks are a terrific form of staying fit for pregnant Mom while spending time with Dad. But, along the same lines, a hike can also be as invigorating, while changing the scenery.

As with any form of exercise, your spouse is going to want to run it by her ob-gyn first. But, if all systems are go, maybe look for a relatively flat trail at a park or in the local mountains or woods. The beauty of a hike is that the two of you are not only away from life's annoyances at home, but also much of modern day Man's disturbances: cars, streets, music, stop lights, etc...

Mom will love spending one-on-one time with you out in nature. You'll both be feeling fit. You'll have peace, as well as time, in which to talk or just be in each other's presence. And, you'll have the opportunity to get back to nature. A good number of women I've spoken with have told me that pregnancy really allowed them to realize that they were part of the big picture. Kelly G. from Kansas told me that no matter how much money a woman has, how big her house is, how extravagant her clothes are, when it comes time to have that baby, she has to push it out like her ancestors thousands of years before her.

So, when a pregnant woman, who feels like she's part of our species' circle of life, is allowed to spend time in the wilderness hiking with the man who helped create her child, she feels closer to him. And, that makes her feel romantic.

"We took evening walks together. These were important for exercise and for talking out the (pregnancy/ birth) process."
-Jen H., California

Share the Written Word

"We would read the pregnancy books together every evening before bed. It was fun to 'oooh' and 'ahhh' over the upcoming changes."
-Julie C., Mom For Seven Months

Time together doesn't always have to be spent focusing on your pregnant partner. No offense, but she's going to need some time to herself, too. One of the most fantastic ways to pull off this seemingly impossible dichotomy is through reading. I'm not talking about reading to each other or sharing a book. I'm just talking about reading together, in proximity.

It's one of the most intimate, non-intimate activities a couple can share. Sit on opposite ends of the couch, allowing your feet to co-mingle, or climb under the sheets together, propped up with pillows, and read together in bed. And, when she laughs, ask her, "What?", and let her tell you. And, when you read something incredible, put your book down and say, "I've got to read something to you."

It sounds so simple, and it is, but it's also terribly effective. She may even comment on the comfort of it all the following day. But, make it a point to try to do it so much that it's almost routine, like saying, "Good morning", or sharing a kiss before you part. Mom will love the closeness of it, while also having her own space.

But, don't stop there. There's also a time and a place to read to each other. If Mom finds an article about pregnancy or birth or babies that she just has to share, drop what you're doing, lie on the floor and listen to it. If you have come across a comic in the Sunday paper that speaks volumes to you, share it with her. Everything you share with one another does not have to revolve around Baby. It can be about the two of you. Remember, you are the foundation of this family unit. That foundation needs to remain strong so that your family will remain strong and sound.

Some couples will share a novel during pregnancy. They choose a book that both partners have wanted to read, and each night they read a portion of it aloud. Maybe one partner will read each evening, or Mom and Dad can alternate reading days. Dad could even read the first half of the book and Mom could read the second.

Sharing a novel together is definitely an exercise in sharing time together as a couple. It's also a lively springboard for conversation. When you read a book together, you feel as though you've just experienced a journey with your partner. It's a hundred times more intense than going to the movies together.

Some couples find solace, comfort and guidance through reading their religion's Holy Scriptures. No matter what you read, or how you go about expressing it, sharing the written word together as a couple can be both intimate and individual; it's warm, and it's more time spent together. So, read.

"He prayed with me and for me."
-Sabina, Overdue

Prepare

"He practiced our relaxation techniques every night."
-S. E., Mom For Three Months

What a splendid way to share in the pregnancy, show your partner some love and spend some quality time together. Any opportunity to be a part of the pregnancy process, pregnant women say, is incredibly romantic. It brings you closer to your partner, and it brings you both closer to Baby. So, take classes together and attend doctor visits with your wife.

So, when Mom suggests a childbirth class, a visit to the maternity ward at the hospital in which she'll be delivering, or a relaxation course, jump on the opportunity to share it with her. Clear your calendar. Leave the cell phone at home. Drop the kids off at the sitter, because this pregnancy will never happen again. This baby is born only once. And, your partner wants you to be a part of it.

But, what will give you even more quality time, and, for many, actually takes more effort than attending class, is practicing at home. When you clear your calendar one-hour a week to learn breathing techniques with a half dozen other pregnant couples, you're showing Mom you care. But, when you make time every evening, regardless of work, TV and emails, to practice what you've learned in class, your relationship grows faster than a dandelion on Miracle-Gro.

This is your time to really put in to practice the positions, the visualization, the patterned breathing, and the focus techniques that seemed so easy with the instructor in the room. Now, you can get a feel for what it's like without help from others, without the opportunity to look at the couple beside you to see if you're doing it right. And, maybe as important, it gives the two of you time to communicate, to stop and discuss what really works for you as a delivery coach and what she finds works best for her as a woman in labor.

You'll find that with every opportunity to spend quality time with the mother of your baby, you'll grow closer to her. She can feel this. That closeness, that growth in emotional proximity, is love manifested and measured in time. Time together, not just next to each other, but really together, is like regular deposits into your romance bank account. You don't realize it at first, but soon you find your bankbook has grown and the deposits become easier, no longer a struggle, financially or emotionally.

"He came to every doctor's visit and avoided leaving town for work."
-Ellie A., From Italy

10 Ways To Enjoy Quality Time With Mom-To-Be

1. Take a nightly walk around the neighborhood. Make it a ritual like brushing your teeth and flushing the toilet.
2. When it's time to prep the nursery, do it together, from discussing the colors, to picking out the furniture, to putting up the border.
3. One of the best places to catch up on the day is in the shower. Shower together as much as possible so you can enjoy Mama's changing body and have uninterrupted time alone.
4. Sign up for birth classes. Attend them. Then, practice what you've learned at home regularly.
5. Go on a drive, not necessarily for the sake of arriving anywhere, but for the drive itself.
6. If Mom wants to shop for baby clothes or toys, join her in the adventure.
7. Take her out to Sunday brunch every now and again. I don't know what it is about combining two meals on Sunday, but for some reason a brunch seems a lot more exciting than either breakfast or lunch.
8. Read books and magazines together about Baby, pregnancy, and childbirth.
9. Drop the kids off at Grandma's and focus on her (your partner, not Grandma). Enjoy her presence. Remember what it's like to be a couple.
10. Listen to her fears and dreams about the coming weeks, months, and years.

"I have to say the most romantic thing was going on our evening walks. It gave us a chance to talk about our future and spend some time away from the distractions of TV and other people."
-Julie, 28 Year-Old Inspector

8

To Give Is Divine

"He gave me a necklace with three garnet hearts - for me, him and the baby. It was romantic because I felt like our relationship was growing in a new direction."

-S. E., 32 Year-Old Teacher

Although a hug, a kind word, or some time together are all fabulous ways to offer romance to your pregnant spouse, let's face it, giving a gift, an actual item, a tangible present is something everyone appreciates, especially Mom-to-be. Coming home to find a bouquet of flowers or the surprise of a handcrafted poem about your relationship are physical representations of your love.

There are a myriad of gifts that Moms-to-be will appreciate and that will make them feel special, cared for and loved. You could thank her with a gift for carrying your child for nine months, or purchase one for labor. Many women feel romanced when Dad-to-be comes home with goodies for Baby. And, a gift that works anytime is one for your spouse, not because she'll be a mom, but because she's the love of your life.

The Landlord Gift

"I loved that my husband brought me a thing that you put in the bathtub that made the water vibrate really hard. It was great for my back. He bought it for my birthday."

-Kristy, Mother of Scott

You know when you're renting a place and you want to make sure the landlord treats you right? You want him to be sure he keeps the rent down and the maintenance up. So, when the holidays role around, you make sure you get him a little something.

Well, Mom-to-be is kind of like the landlord to your child. Baby is just borrowing the space for a bit, and Mom is in charge of its upkeep and repairs. Granted, you don't have to bribe Mom to be sure she stays healthy for herself and the baby. But, like a landlord that you appreciate and respect, you might offer her a gift of thanks for doing a bang-up job.

A water massager is a gift that says, "Thank you for protecting and sheltering our baby." It shows a woman that her hard work and the discomfort she's experiencing is appreciated. When we, as men, can express our appreciation for Mom's pregnancy, she feels acknowledged and loved.

A poem or a love letter about her strength during these nine months, about how great a mom she already is, or about how well she's been caring for Baby en-utero is a heartfelt gift Mom will cherish. Type it up or have it written professionally in calligraphy. Then, frame it. This is a gift from the soul that will stand the test of time.

When you attend your twenty week ob-gyn visit, the one with the ultrasound, arrange it with Doc beforehand that she stick an extra ultrasound picture aside and slip it to you when Mom is taking one of her seven trips per hour to the bathroom. Then, head over to your local frame shop and find one that has baby items surrounding the glass (blocks, Teddy Bears, etc...). Then, leave it on the bathroom counter by the sink for her to find before you head off to work.

When my wife, Mary, was pregnant with our first child, I searched our music collection for songs about babies, children, moms, and parenthood. I compiled the songs I found (Stevie Wonder's "Isn't She Lovely", Peaches & Herb's "One Child Of Love", as well as comedy snippets about parenthood from Ellen DeGeneres and Bill Cosby) and presented the tape to her for being such an awesome home for our baby.

Along the same lines, find a song that represents how you feel about your spouse during this pregnancy (Bette Midler's "Wind Beneath My Wing" or Stevie Wonder's "You Are the Sunshine of My

Life") and dedicate it to her on your local radio station when you know she'll be listening. The romantic results will quadruple if her friends, family or co-workers also hear the dedication. Although most men prefer to keep their attempts at romance highly classified secrets, many women tend to appreciate public romantic efforts. They not only show your significant other that she's cared for, but that you have no problem professing it to the world. So, a public song dedication, as is being suggested here, can really turn on those romance faucets.

"He bought me new computer games once in awhile so I could have something new to play during those middle-of-the-night, can't sleep hours when my body was so uncomfortable I had to get out of bed."
-Arizona D., Teacher

Labor Day Presents

"He bought me gifts for labor: my favorite candies and an exercise ball."
-Jen, Former Teacher

Jen's husband is a wise man. When Mom goes into labor, you want to make her as happy and as comfortable as you possibly can. Although there's only so much you can do about her physical discomfort, emotionally, you can be the one who's "thought of everything."

Buy some gifts before labor that you think she may appreciate while Baby is making his debut. The exercise ball (for birthing on) and any favorite treat she may crave (although many women lose their appetite during labor) are excellent delivery gifts.

You may also want to purchase a wooden back roller or an electronic massager to relieve back and neck tension or for counter pressure purposes. The idea for a special compilation of songs put on a tape or CD as previously mentioned, can be a great gift to play during delivery. Or maybe you could purchase that soothing classical CD or the tape of relaxing ocean sounds she's been talking about getting, but never finding the time to buy.

If you haven't already given her the framed ultrasound photo, presenting it during delivery as a point of focus can be extremely meaningful, and inspirational. Some women have difficulty focusing on the end result during delivery. They only know that with each contraction they are experiencing discomfort. They can easily forget that there is an end, and that end is a new life. By having a photo of that end result, framed and staring her in the face, Mom may be able to hang tougher and longer through the difficult contractions.

But, don't forget that Mom needs romance after labor, too. All too often, after Mom gives her final push, all the focus is on this incredible new life in the world, as well it should be. If you're prepared, focus can still be on Baby, but Mom can share in it.

Prepare a gift that speaks volumes. Flowers are pretty. A teddy bear is cute. But, we're talking about depth here. This woman just pushed a living creature into the world. What is it that truly represents the past nine months you two have gone through, the delivery you just experienced, the thankfulness for carrying your baby, the pride you have in your partner?

Find or make a creative and specific gift, and give it to the mother of your baby. It doesn't have to be elaborate or expensive. If it comes from the heart and expresses your feelings, she will cherish it, and you, for years to come.

"He bought me half carat diamond earrings as a 'thank you' for the physical discomfort and pain I endured during pregnancy, which I still wear everyday (even though our daughter is almost fourteen)."
-Valerie, 46 Year-Old Manager

Something For the Little One

"One of the main things that my husband has done so far that I thought was so special was he got our unborn daughter a couple of Christmas presents and had me open them. He totally did it on his own. I didn't even know he was going to. I was just so touched that he did that, and, to me, it was totally romantic."
-Nicole, Age 30

When you bring a gift home for your "little one," you tend to trigger an emotional switch in Mom-to-be. By coming home with a present for the baby you've never met, you're showing Mom that you are a caring and nurturing father. This gives her confidence in the selection of a mate and father for her baby. If you are willing to offer gifts to unborn Baby, you must be a protecting and providing man. This increases Mom's serotonin levels, which leads to feelings of love and romance.

Although some women may not say so outright, most want a partner they can feel safe with, one whom they have complete confidence will raise and love their offspring. If you are that man, you are bringing romance to the table of your relationship every day of every week of every month of her pregnancy.

So, head on over to the local baby shop and pick up an educational block that plays Beethoven when it's jostled. Or, make a beeline to the infant section of your local department store and get a onesie with your wife's favorite color on it. I remember seeing a matching Los Angeles Lakers basketball team jersey and shorts for a one-year old when my wife was pregnant with our first child. She found it so endearing that I purchased the set without even knowing the baby's gender. I told her, regardless if it's a boy or a girl, the baby will be wearing this outfit one day as we watch the Lakers' games together.

There are hundreds, maybe even thousands of gifts you can bring home for Baby that will make Mom feel even closer to you: lullaby CD, board book, video, a cute bib, first shoes, blankets. The list goes on. But you can also offer gifts that come less from the store and more from the heart. A beautiful keepsake your child will cherish and Mom will melt for is a video diary of the pregnancy with interviews from Mom and Dad, as well as siblings and grandparents. It can be used to document doctor visits, Mom's growing tummy, the first kicks, and all the incredible experiences you'd love to share with your little one. (One recommendation, though: after Baby's born, edit your nine month record down to the most exciting and poignant moments, to make watching the tape a treat rather than a chore.)

You can also write Baby a letter, or letters, while you're waiting to meet her. Tell her how you found out Mom was pregnant. Share your feelings about the pregnancy and the anticipation building toward the big day. You can mention how Baby's name was chosen and what was going on in the world as Baby was developing in Mama. Save the letters until your offspring has matured enough to appreciate them. Not only will your child enjoy your letters, but Mom will feel a strong attraction to you as you write them, then again, years later, as you offer them to your child.

If you want to do something personal for your child, but you're neither a filmmaker nor a writer, how about a time capsule? Head to your local toy store and buy a handful of the most popular toys. Put them in a box. Throw in the newspaper of the day your wife delivers. Then, stick it all aside for twenty years. Spring it out one day and show your now adult-child what was popular and what was going on when she was born. The effort you put into a project like this will bring your partner and your child closer to you than you can imagine.

"He went shopping one day on his own and came home with darling pajamas for the baby. It was fun to see him excited about our child-to-be and to know he was dreaming about the day the baby would wear the PJ's."

-Cathi S., Teacher

Because It's Her

"He could have brought me some little token of affection (like a candy bar, soda, flowers, cards, peanuts, anything) that would have let me know he was thinking of me."
                              -A. D., Age 31

That's right, A. D., we've been thinking of Baby and Mom-to-be, but what about the woman in the midst of all of this? No, not the pregnant lady. Not the soon-to-be mother. But, the woman you fell in love with. She's still there. Although during this time so much is about the baby and the pregnancy and the delivery, take time out not for Mom, but for your partner. Let her know that you appreciate her for her.

Think back to pre-pregnancy days. You may have to go back a bit farther, but think about the times when you were romantic with your partner for the sake of romance. What surprises did you bring home to her? What gifts did you make? Did you write her poetry or leave her love notes on the bathroom mirror? Did you surprise her with jewelry or her favorite perfume?

Did you slip conversation hearts into her sack lunch? And, what about outfits? Forty-eight year old, family educator, Tracy Schmidt announces, "Buy her a surprise, cute (sexy) dress or undies from the maternity shops."

And, what woman doesn't love chocolate? Chocolate, especially dark chocolate, is chock full of phenylethylamine, a chemical that makes us feel the same way we do when we're in love. So, bring home a candy bar now and again. And, don't worry about ill effects on Baby's health. Researchers at the University of Helsinki found that babies born to women who ate chocolate daily during pregnancy laughed and smiled more at six months than babies whose mothers fought the urge to satisfy their sweet tooth.

"Buy us nice bath bubbles."
-Rebecca, Manager from the U.K.

9 Gifts to Bring Home During Pregnancy

1. Anything associated with massage: electric massager, back roller, massage oil (But you also have to deliver the massage).
2. A gift certificate to a clothing store to pick out a cute outfit. A gift certificate is always a safe bet when it comes to buying pregnant women clothing, but be sure you attend the shopping excursion so you can add your two cents.
3. An outfit for Baby. This does not need to be a gift certificate; just be sure it's easy on the eyes. Always ask advice from the person at the register if you're unsure.
4. Flowers. It's nearly impossible to go wrong with this romantic staple.
5. Make a tape for Mom with all her favorite songs on it. She can use it during the evening walks, or make one with relaxation sounds: waves, rain, even Bach. She may want to play it during breathing practice or during delivery.
6. Write a letter to your baby and stash it away for him.
7. Jewelry is another gift that's difficult to mess up. One mom told me that she appreciated receiving necklaces because they would bring attention to her face rather than the changing body she was uncomfortable with.
8. Frame the ultrasound picture, and surprise Mom-to-be with it.
9. Create a poem for Mom about how great a woman she is and a mom she will be.

"Little gifts and surprises would have been a nice touch. I guess my husband had his own insecurities about being a dad. Thus, he literally didn't really start to get excited about Baby until the ninth month. Only then he started to buy me and the baby little gifts."
-A. C., 38 Year-Old Manager

9

Take A Load Off

"I wish he would have done more of the house duties for me. There's nothing more romantic when you're pregnant than a husband taking on more responsibility (without being asked). Even when you're not pregnant, a man with a mop in his hands IS sexy."
-Debbie S., Mother of Two

So, go ahead, give her a thrill, a mop in one hand, a vacuum in the other, Debbie's dream guy. In all seriousness, though, nearly one out of every five women surveyed said they found it romantic when their men took the initiative to help out around the house.

It may not look like it, but that woman carrying your child is working tremendously hard, every minute, every day, for forty weeks. She needs to eat more because she burns more calories. She needs more sleep because she's expending more energy, living for two. Do her a favor, and take some of the load off of her shoulders.

I've passed this advice on to many men, and there are those who'd rather have back-to-back root canals than clean a toilet bowl or dust end tables. But a wise man will take it all in stride, like Peter Greenberg of Connecticut did when his wife was pregnant: "I didn't particularly like the extra housework, but I didn't fight it." Smart fellow.

How *can* you fight it, anyway? It's not as though Mom-to-be is suddenly using pregnancy as an excuse to opt out of keeping the house together. Chances are, if she could, she'd rather fold the laundry and feed the cats, because you don't have the "knack" she does. But, since she's busy using her energy to keep your baby healthy and growing, she'll allow you the honor of the housework.

So, try to step up and into Mom's shoes for a few months. If you see something's not getting done, try doing it yourself. Don't know how? Not an excuse. Ask.

Take off the old toilet paper roll and replace it with a new one. What, no TP in the bathroom?! Replenish the supply.

Finding little chunks of food and grains of sand embedded in you shoulder after you get up from watching a TV show from the floor? Vacuum the living room.

Looking through your closet all you find is a pair of mismatched socks, BVD's that look more like Swiss cheese than undergarments, pants with a waist four inches smaller than yours, and a shirt that would be great at an 80's theme party. Time to do the laundry. Separate like colors and whites. Use the correct settings. And, when everything's clean and dry, fold, iron, and put away.

A man can only live on a jar of olives and a half container of peanut butter for only so long. Besides, you always need to have an ample supply of nutritious foods for Mom in the house. So, go shopping. Don't just head out with a credit card and crossed fingers. Look through your fridge, cabinets, and pantry. Make a list of your regular items that are low or out. Ask your partner for some help here. When you return, put away the groceries. By the way, not everything fits in the fridge. Use the cabinets, too.

Basically, Mom wants you to fill in where she's lacking. She probably won't ask you to take on the entire household chore repertoire, but there are two main areas that pregnant moms request the most help: dishes and dinner. If you could lift the burden in just these two areas, in her eyes you'd go from Don King to Don Juan in the romance department.

"I wish he'd pitched in with the chores more."
-Tracy, Age 28 From North Carolina

Experience Dishpan Hands

"I loved falling asleep on the couch at around 9:00 at night, after putting our toddler to bed and waking to hear him doing dishes. I

knew he was doing them to help me. In letting me sleep and caring about my workload, I felt so loved."

-Cathi, 32 Year-Old Homemaker

The Dreaded Dishes, every husband's biggest fear. And, it doesn't matter who you are, there's something about that pile of soiled plates and bowls that make even the manliest man cringe. For many of us when we see that Mt. Everest of dirty Corning Ware and coffee-stained mugs, we suddenly imagine we're playing Jenga, "I think I can balance the saucer between the frying pan and the soup ladle without an avalanche occurring." And, if the pile stays steady for five seconds or more, we're off the dishwashing hook.

It's our partners who usually find our "towers" and end up demolishing them, cleaning each individual building block, and setting them in the dish rack to dry. Sure, we get off without washing the dishes, but at the expense of romance.

Now that your partner is expecting, you need to avoid the dish towers. We men know that women would appreciate it if we took control of the dish situation. If you have a dishwasher, load it, turn it on, and unload it. If you don't have one, buy one. If you can't buy one, wash the dishes by hand.

Pregnancy can be a stressful time in a woman's life. When you pick up the pieces, like washing the dishes, you're meeting the needs of your partner. She feels safe and cared for because of your actions. When a woman feels protected and that her needs are being met, the levels of the neurotransmitter, serotonin, increase. With increased serotonin levels your partner can begin experiencing lower levels of stress and anxiety. She can begin to see the trees and not just the forest. She becomes positive and optimistic. Her brain releases endorphins, and she's a happy woman. She feels loved, all due to some Palmolive and a pair of rubber gloves.

"He did the dishes for me because 'my tummy was in the way'. For him, that was romantic."

-Stephanie W., Stay At Home Mom

You've Gotta Eat

"I wish he would have cooked more often during the later months. Planning and preparing all the meals really became a chore the further along the pregnancy went."
-Monica M., Office Manager

Of all the household chores pregnant women have told me they wished their partners would take over, cooking meals was number one. I don't know if it's because they get to be off their tired feet, or if all the aromas cause them to lose their appetites, or if it's merely a matter of one less thing to prepare and plan for. Regardless of the reason, passing the cooking apron to their men ranks at the top of pregnant women's lists. So, we might as well aim to please.

Think about how stressed this pregnancy is making you: more financial obligations, prepping the nursery, what will the baby be like, will it be healthy, breastfeed or bottle. Now, take that anxiety and multiply in by 412. That's the level of stress at which Mom-to-be is surviving. She doesn't get a break from pregnancy. She can't walk away from it. She feels the kicks in her sleep. She realizes the changes when she showers. At work and at the store, everyone asks about the pregnancy. At breakfast she's nauseated. During sex her positioning is limited. There is no escape. So, when anxiety sets in, any help is appreciated.

Therefore, it's time to open *The Joy of Cooking* and see what you can whip up. You might want to ask Mom-to-be what she's in the mood for, or, if you have a knack in the kitchen, surprise her with a special dish. No matter what you cook, odds are your partner will appreciate it. Maybe it's because she gets to relax while it's simmering. Maybe it's the anticipation of the meal, but for some reason, when someone else cooks, the food often tastes better.

Don't forget, though, if you have other children, you need to cook for them, too. To save you from overworking yourself, cook one dish, something for Mom and the kids. But, be sure you're preparing nutritious meals. Boxed or fried foods are often easy to prepare, but you must remember, you're not only feeding your partner, but your developing child, also. Whatever Mama eats, Baby eats. So, keep it healthy.

Now, when dinner's done, you have to clear the table and wash the dishes. If you leave this for her, dinner is no longer a relaxing meal. It's the quiet before the cleaning storm. To really make the dinner experience a romantic one, women tell me that we men need to be in charge of it from the first cracked egg, to the cleaning of the last teaspoon. If you've already got little ones running around the house, enlist them as your clean-up crew.

If you don't have your own crew, you don't have time to do the dishes, or you can't cook your way out of a wet macaroni and cheese box, don't fret. You can still be your pregnant partner's hero. "How?" you ask. It's called "take-out".

Call a local restaurant and place an order to pick up after work. Or, call a delivery service from home and get door-to-door service. The perks: save precious time, no fear of ruining the meal, and all the china and silverware are disposable. Once again, though, order something tasty but also nutritious for the love of your life and the life that you love.

"Sometimes I'm so tired, I can hardly stand it, and when he steps in and does little things to help out, I appreciate it tremendously. One night he made dinner, for example. And, he doesn't cook. So it meant so much. I was taking a nap, and when I woke up, dinner was almost cooked. I think we just appreciate being taken care of."
-Sarah, Pregnant

10 Ways to Ease Her Load

1. Do the grocery shopping.
2. Sort, wash, dry, and fold the laundry.
3. Balance the checkbook, and keep up on the bills.

4. Wash her car.
5. Vacuum, sweep, and mop now and again.
6. Wash and stow away the dishes.
7. Gas her car for her.
8. Iron.
9. Cook the meals.
10. And, remember, if you do it wrong, she'll still appreciate the
        attempt. Effort truly does go a long way in a relationship.

"I really wish he had done more around the house when I was so tired. That would be the most romantic thing he could have done."
                    -S. E., 38 Year-Old New Mom

10

Encore

"The most romantic thing my husband ever did for me was to take care of our children for a few hours so I could have a break. It gave me time to pamper myself, read, or just get some much needed rest. Afterwards, I was always much more relaxed and much 'friendlier' towards him."

-Jen C., 29 Year-Old Mother of Four

For a first-time dad-to-be, pregnancy can be one of life's most exciting mysteries. Everything is so incredible: the staggering concept of conception, the realization that two lives have created a third, hearing your baby's heartbeat for the first time, understanding that the bump in your wife's tummy is your growing child, accepting the fact that you're no longer just some guy, but somebody's father. It can all be a bit overwhelming, emotional, and exhilarating.

But when it comes to a second, third, or even sixth pregnancy, for some dads, the novelty has worn off. It no longer feels like a magical experience, but merely a familiar process, a formality that must be endured to get a baby. The two of you have already done this. You know what to expect. It's no longer about the two of you focusing on this baby. Now, you've got a family to take care of: play dates to fill, bedtime stories to read, babysitters to pay, and sleep to catch up on. You just can't focus on the pregnancy as you did the first time around.

You don't have to. But you do have to focus on it, on her, on the baby. Even though you've been through it once, twice, or eight times already, each pregnancy renders a different experience. It's like going fishing. You'll never forget the first time you reeled in a fish on your own. You'd never experienced such a rush before: the feel of the first nibble, the sight of your bob dipping its head, and the thrill of finally getting a look at the fish you landed.

Although you've already caught a fish, you return to go at it again. Why? Because now you know a little more than you did the first time. You know what to expect. Yet, the unexpected is what you know you'll experience. The next time you may try different bait or fish at a new spot. It may take longer to hook the fish. The fish may be a different type or different size.

You return to what you know because you know it. Fishing is not an all or nothing sport. You're always in a process of bettering yourself, of learning. And, like pregnancy, you use what you've learned to better handle what you haven't yet experienced.

The Novelty Has Worn Off

"My husband would sing songs and tell stories to my belly when we were pregnant with our son and daughter. I felt that although my body was changing daily, he was still connected with me and just as excited about meeting our babies as I was."
-D. S., Age 31

Some second round pops aren't as enthused with the process as D. S.'s husband. Conception is great. Can't wait for the baby to arrive. But, pregnancy just isn't as exciting. These men are less involved because they know what to expect. They may also feel less anxious about their partner's and their baby's health, having already gone through pregnancy before. Well, these dads need to realize that although it's not new, each pregnancy is novel. And, pregnant partners need as much TLC, as much attention, and as much romance as they received during pregnancy number one. Just because she's already gone through it before, doesn't mean she doesn't need a shoulder massage this pregnancy, or doesn't desire to be told she's gorgeous, or want you to be her support, her Superman, again.

Mom doesn't want to have to go through the process alone. So, like pregnancy number one, your partner would probably love for you to accompany her to her doctor's appointments, attend childbirth refresher classes with her, help create a baby name list, and go layette and nursery shopping with her.

And, keep in mind, although you have experienced a pregnancy, each one is different, even within the same woman. And, each one is just as important as the last. Also, with each pregnancy, romance can change, too.

Allison Stiles, of South Portland, Maine, felt voluptuous, attractive, and very sexy during her first pregnancy. She marveled in her changing self and basked in the feeling. But, during pregnancy number two, it "...didn't go fast enough. I was bored and miserable to be around." Instead of a titanic libido, as in pregnancy number one, Allison described sensations as "prickly". She just wasn't comfortable in her body, and therefore was very frustrated.

As a partner, you must adapt to each pregnancy. You have to be a chameleon. When she changes, so must you, so as to keep romance alive. If you are unsure of how to change, what angle to approach her, first try to read her. But, when all else fails (or even before "when all else fails"), communicate. Ask her what she needs, wants and desires. Just you asking during the second or third pregnancy demonstrates to her that you value her, her baby, and her pregnancy even when you've been through it before. That value is read as love.

Take the Kids... Please

"I wish he'd let me sleep while he watched the older children."
-Tracy S., Retail Work

Pregnant moms who already had children told me time and again, the same thing, "Helping me with the children really showed me he cared." When it was just you, your partner, and a pregnant belly, you could focus your efforts directly toward Mom-to-be. But, now that there is already the pitter-patter of little feet around the house, Mom needs your help more than ever, because not only is there a pregnancy to deal with, but there's also the family.

Mom must deal with the pregnancy. She can't escape it for nine months. So, that leaves the family in your hands. Most moms I spoke with weren't asking for seclusion from the rest of the family until Baby was born. Instead, they wanted Dad to take charge and give Mom the time and space she needed to revitalize, reenergize, and regain her sanity.

So, how can you fulfill Mom's wishes? Overwhelmingly moms are asking for breaks from the kids. Send her out for time away from sibling battles, tantrums, and diaper changes. Although she can't escape pregnancy, allow your partner to escape the stresses that family life can sometimes bring.

It will definitely be a challenge for you, but your partner will appreciate it. Send her to the spa for a day, a makeover, a manicure and pedicure. Tell her you'll take care of this, and she should go out to lunch and shopping by herself or with a friend. Encourage her to have a girls' day or evening out. They could all catch a movie or go out to dinner.

Your encouragement alone will be appreciated more than you can imagine. Then, when she comes back, you're bound to see a new woman, one who has "juiced up", who's had a bit of time away and is now reenergized to continue on. Taking on the task of manning the home alone is definitely a challenge for many dads, but the results are well worth it, not only for Mom, but for the dynamics of the entire family; besides, it's incredibly romantic.

If Mom's unable to get away from the stresses of family by going out, let her stay home, and take the family away from her. Head to a park. Go bowling. Spend the day at the beach. And, let Mom have the house to herself with no crying, diapers, screaming, or squabbles to squelch. Just a day to enjoy a soothing bath or read a magazine, or catch up on her sleep, or watch her favorite video, or to work in the garden.

It really doesn't matter what she does, as long as she gets the opportunity to decide in a peaceful home. An added romantic touch would be to leave something behind for her to entice her to enjoy her peace: bath oils, a relaxing CD, lunch delivered.

And, when life is too busy to be able to pack up the kids or allow Mom to sneak away, take up the slack at home. Help with the kids' homework. Change the diapers. Make sack lunches for school. Give the kids their baths. Prepare the meals. This is what pregnant Moms who already have children say will make them feel special and cared for.

They say it's the little things that make the biggest difference. If Mom's in the bathroom with the door closed, don't let Junior disturb her. On Sunday morning if Mom's sleeping in, and the kids are up, shut the bedroom door so she can sleep longer. When the toddler calls, "Mommy!" at 3:00 in the morning, pull your feet out of bed and deal with it so Mommy can get a decent night's sleep.

Keep in mind that morning sickness can increase in times of stress (i. e., screaming rug rats), back pain gets worse when Mom's constantly lifting or carrying the children, and fatigue is a huge factor when little ones continually rely on Mom. You must step in and relieve Mom. You can even get older children to help out. Not only are they out of the way and not vying for Mom's attention, but they're helping to relieve the load she feels she must bear.

You can't do it all, but any help with the kids, Moms say, really takes the edge off. So, step up and be her Man of Steel. You can do it. These kids are just flesh and bone, no kryptonite added.

"He bought me a certificate for a day spa, which meant I got a day alone without our toddler, and he encouraged me to pamper myself while pregnant."

-C. S., Mother of Two

Something For The Ones Already Here

"He could have cooked nourishing meals for the family so I did not have to work so much at my job and at home."
                    -T. S., 28 Year-Old Full Time Mom

As far as romance, the focus of this book has been on what Dad-to-be can say or do for Mom-to-be. Another way to touch Mom is by circumventing her altogether. The target: your current children.

Since your partner has been pregnant, a lot of the focus that was once bestowed upon your current little ones has been geared toward Mom, or the nursery, or the new baby clothes and toys. And, after baby arrives, even more attention will be lavished on the new bundle of joy, which can leave some children feeling frustrated and jealous.

Before Baby arrives, make a conscious effort to spend quality time with your children without mentioning the new baby or Mommy's big tummy. Let your children know how truly cherished they are.

You might even want to create something for your current child by yourself, or with him, that symbolizes the special bond that the two of you have and that nothing and nobody (not even a eight pound squishy baby) can ever damage. Maybe you can put together a collage of photos of the two of you or of activities you do together. Maybe you can build a tree house together or a model car or airplane.

For my daughter, I sifted through twenty-two hours of home video footage and put together a video of our years before Baby arrived, all to the Lee Ann Womack song, "I Hope You Dance". The last shot is of the two of us dancing when she was a few weeks old, and a message from me: "If you ever need a dance partner, you know where to find me. Dad."

What makes something like this so unforgettable is not only that your child feels cared for and loved and knows that will never change even after Baby arrives, but Mom sees your love for her child, which sparks her maternal instincts. She realizes how great a dad you are, and how great a dad you'll be again with the incoming offspring. When a woman knows her man is taking care of her children, she feels safe and cared for.

"He could have helped with the other kids and the housework."
-Jodi, Age 34

10 Ways to Make "The Next" Pregnancy Easy For Her

1. Cook breakfast on the weekends while Mom sleeps in.
2. Take the children miniature golfing.
3. Arrange for your child to have a sleepover at a friend's house.
4. Make it a house rule: "When Mom's in the bathroom, she is not to be disturbed." Then, enforce it.
5. Pick the kids up from their games. Drop them off at school.
6. Change the baby's diapers.
7. Take childbirth classes again. Guaranteed, you'll pick up something you didn't get the first, second, or fifth time.
8. Teach the kids how to set and clear the table.
9. Try to keep the noise level to a low rumble.
10. Do whatever it takes to make each pregnancy unique.

Week-By-Week Romance Suggestions

What I've learned about men and romance through my seminars is that, although many of us have our hearts in the right places, we fall back into our old patterns quickly unless we're given specific means to avoid that pitfall.

At my seminars men would talk about what romance was and what women found romantic. We'd share success stories of romance as well as nightmares of failed attempts at romance. We'd watch clips from movies, listen to romantic songs, practice writing love letters and poems, discuss the most romantic restaurants and spots in town.

The men would leave all pumped up and ready to sweep their partners off their feet. Then, a week later, they'd start trickling in... the emails: "Okay, what was it again you said that chocolate does to a woman's brain chemistry?", "What were those three things to do that make any moment romantic?", "You told us a simple way to get ourselves out of the doghouse. What was it again?"

It wasn't until I added a simple page to my folder of handouts that the problem all but disappeared. It was a page that listed "50 Simple Romantic Gestures." I told men to refer to it, to do one a day starting with number one. When they got to number fifty, it was time to start back at the top of the list again. By the end of the year, they would have gone through the list seven times, and romance would be alive in their homes. And, it was.

Very often we men need more specifics to apply the theoretical information we're so excited about putting to the test.

So, the following three chapters are a week-by-week list of romantic ideas for men to consider while their partners are with child. The chapters are broken down by trimesters, and each week's idea comes straight from a woman who's been there and is offered for that specific week based on Mom's physical, biological, and physiological changes due to her pregnancy.

You should not feel compelled to *have to* do anything precisely how it's been laid out. Each pregnancy, each woman, each relationship, and each couple is different. Let the following ideas inspire you. Use them how they're presented, change them to fit your situation or switch them around based on your partner's needs. But, whatever you decide, do something. This pregnancy is only going to happen once.

11

Trimester One: The Queasy Months

The first trimester is an incredible time full of excitement and anxiety. After discovering that you two are expecting, it's a terrific opportunity to wonder: will it be a boy or a girl, what name will you give the baby, will it look like you or more like Mom, how will this child affect the world?

Along with dreaming about the future, you'll need to also focus on the present. And, your here-and-now attention needs to be aimed at your pregnant partner. Although she's still going to want to be romanced, this is when you'll need to change things up a bit. Just because your partner's not showing doesn't mean she's not changing.

When attempting to be romantic with your partner, keep in mind what's going on during this first trimester. Many women experience nausea and/or morning sickness at the beginning of their pregnancies. There's bound to be emotional and hormonal adjustments. So, you'll have to be patient and develop a thick skin. And, because her body is creating the placenta, the baby's life support system, she may become easily fatigued during these first few months. She may require an extra one to two hours of sleep per day.

If she's not too tired or emotional, and is well rested, you may consider sexual intimacy. But, keep in mind that those enlarged breasts are tender right about now. And, don't be surprised if she needs to interrupt the passion with a trip to the ladies' room. Frequent urination is very common this first part of pregnancy. That said, here are some romantic suggestions Mom might appreciate:

(Weeks 1-5) The Buds of New Life

Materials:
• six to twelve red roses

• one single rose (or other flower) of another color

"When I found out I was pregnant with our oldest daughter, my husband sent me flowers at work. There were six red roses for me and, in the middle of them, there was one yellow (my favorite rose) for the baby! I had been trying to get pregnant after a miscarriage and he did this knowing how much it meant as the yellow rose is so special to me. I had lost my dad to cancer one and a half years earlier, and my mom told me a special story that concerned her and my dad and yellow roses, and my husband remembered the story, He made sure to put that yellow rose in the middle of the red roses. He was so sweet, and I think that was the most special thing he ever could have done for me. I love him so much for it, and he, to this day, is the world's best dad."

-Michelle R., Indiana Mommy

What to do:

Each couple discovers that they're pregnant in different ways and at different times. Some women know immediately... intuitively. Some men can detect it right away, too. There are couples that won't suspect it until she misses a period. Still, others are unaware of the pregnancy until the third month.

No matter how and when you discover you're going to be a daddy, one way to show your excitement, to say thank you, and to express your love is through a bouquet of roses.

The week you learn your spouse is pregnant, surprise her with a bouquet of red roses, or any other flowers she may love. Let her know that these flowers represent the love you have for her. Then, in the midst of these, have one single flower standing out. I like the idea of it being a bud that will bloom in a day or two. You can pick her favorite color, a significant color, or a neutral color like yellow because the baby's gender is still unknown.

The bud represents the new life that will be blooming in your lives, surrounded by a sea of your love, the love that created it.

(Week 6) The Apple (Seed) of Your Eye

Materials:
• apple or orange or watermelon seeds, or marbles, or Tic-Tacs, etc...
• sealable snack bags
• permanent pen

"I would say things like, 'The baby is only about the size of an apple seed.' And, the next day, he brought me home some apple seeds from work in a little plastic bag with a date on it. It let me know that he listened to me, and thought about the baby even when he was away from me."

-Angela L. Realtor

What to do:
This week, or any during this first trimester, as you read the pregnancy books with your spouse or after she's read to you from a maternity magazine, take note of the size of the embryo that's attached to her uterine wall. Now, go out and find an item of about the same size. Put it in the plastic bag, and put the day's date on it.

You and your partner will both marvel at the size of the small life you've created. It would be such a thoughtful keepsake to look back on after Baby arrives and to think, "You were actually this small." But, most of all, your partner will feel loved, because you're thinking of her and the baby, even when you're not with them.

(Week 7) With a Twist of Lemon

Materials:
• glass of water or cup of tea
• paper towel or washcloth
• a bathroom

"The most romantic thing my husband did for me while I was pregnant was that he would be home when I came home from work with the bathroom door open and a glass of water with lemon in it."
-Paula, Age 29

What to do:

If your spouse is one of the 70% of women who suffer from morning sickness during pregnancy, the good news is it probably will only last a couple more months. The bad news is, you've got to deal with it for a couple more months.

This week start giving your wife moral support when the morning sickness takes over. Be available. Rub her back. Offer her a towel for clean up. And, have a cracker and a glass of water with lemon or a cup of tea available for her when the ordeal is over.

(Week 8) Fill 'Er Up

Materials:
• partner's low gas tank
• gas card, credit card, or cash

"He could have made sure my car was kept filled with gas. I got sick for the first four and a half months of my pregnancy, and this was not a task that was enjoyable."
-Chris M., Independent Business Owner

What to do:

A pregnant woman in her first trimester is often fatigued. She also may have strong aversions to tastes and to smells such as gasoline. And, if she's nauseous on top of all that, you filling up her gas tank is like a gift from the gods.

Starting this week, periodically check her tank level. If it drops below half, run her car over to the station and fill it up. Your act of kindness will allow her to rest, as well as avoid getting unnecessarily sick. A small gesture from you, a huge relief for her.

(Week 9) Smile for the Birdie

Materials:
• camera
• photo albums or frames

"He took pictures of me at different stages of pregnancy and put the pictures up around the house."
                                        -Jen, 27 Year-Old, Stay At Home Mom

What to do:
        Starting this week, take photos of your spouse regularly. You might even want to be sure she poses in ways that show off her tummy. I know of some couples that will take a weekly photo with Mom holding a sign with the date or how many weeks left until Baby arrives.
        What you can do is display the framed photos up around your house or put them in a small photo album in chronological order, so you and your spouse can see the gradual progression and tummy growth through the pregnancy.
        With you taking regular photos of your spouse, she will feel that you find her attractive. And, if she feels attractive during these forty weeks, you've brought romance to your relationship.

<u>(Week 10) Breakfast Is Served</u>

Materials:
• nutritious breakfast foods (e.g. fruits, eggs, juices, beans, yogurt, etc...)

"I was exhausted and sickish during my second pregnancy. Before my husband would leave for work, he'd make me some scrambled eggs with cheese on top and sautéed greens or a scrambled egg burrito, my breakfast of choice at the time, and leave them on a warm plate covered in foil so I could eat something tasty and nourishing before I got out of bed. I felt very loved by this and was the envy of my also-pregnant-at-the-time girlfriends."

-Judith S., Small Business Co-Owner

What to do:
Although many women experience food aversions and morning sickness during their first trimester of pregnancy, others will have healthy appetites. And, if you can find the one meal or two that doesn't cause her to rush to the bathroom, make it for her.

Starting this week, and while she's feeling lethargic, as often as you can, try and make her a nutritious breakfast of foods that she can keep down. If you can bring it to her in bed, that will allow her to conserve her energy while getting some extra sleep. If you must leave before she wakes up, leave it for her in foil or easily microwaved.

She'll definitely appreciate your thoughtfulness, not having to expend extra energy, and being sure that the meal is healthy allows her to know that you are looking out for her and the baby's well being.

(Week 11) Just Say It

Materials:
• a working mouth

"I wish my husband would have taken the time to tell me he loved me more. I feel that pregnancy is a very emotional time, and I think it would have made me feel better."
-Brooke, Age 33

What to do:
Brooke got it dead on. Pregnancy is a very emotional time, and during the first trimester hormones are going off like fireworks at the finale of an Independence Day celebration. Letting your partner know that she's loved, not just through actions, but through words won't tame the hormonal roller coaster, but it will help to curb the dips and curves.

If you haven't made a point to profess your love daily to the woman holding your child, start this week. Tell her every morning when you wake up and every night before you go to sleep. Tell her every time you have to leave. Leave it on the answering machine. Email her. Write it on a stickie and pop it into her planner. Then, after Baby is born, continue! Never miss an opportunity to tell your partner she's the love of your life.

(Week 12) Nighty-Night

Materials:
• a bed
• pillows (preferably a body pillow)
• blanket and/or sheets
• glass of water
• prenatal vitamins

"I would have liked my husband to tuck me into bed, make sure I had my body pillows adjusted and water by the bed."

-Christine, 34 Year-Old, Mother of One

What to do:

Do you remember the comfort you felt when your parents would tuck you in to bed or bring you a glass of water for the bedside? Neither the tuck nor the water really made bedtime more pleasant. It was knowing that someone was there for you, trying to comfort you, fulfilling your requests. You felt safe and provided for. You felt loved.

During pregnancy your partner wants to feel safe and provided for. She wants to feel loved. So, this week, and continuing throughout the pregnancy, start a new nightly ritual. Fluff her pillows. She may start to feel more comfortable sleeping on her side. A body pillow allows her to support her body in comfort. If you don't have a body pillow, offer pillows for her back and between her legs.

Then, don't forget to have a full glass of water for her in case she feels parched during the night. And, if you could help her with her prenatal vitamin by having one on her nightstand next to her water every evening, her, and the baby's, well-being will be much healthier. Oh, and don't forget the goodnight kiss before you turn out the lights.

(Week 13) Let Her Soak

Materials:
• bathtub
• candles
• matches
• reading material (poetry, novel, magazine)

"He got me in the tub - just warm enough - lit candles and read me all sorts of poets."
-Eliza, Photographer

What to do:

A soak in the tub seems to wash away the stresses of the day. For a pregnant woman, it also allows her a time and place to relax. She can ease the swelling in her feet and find time just for herself.

This week, pick an evening and draw your partner a warm bath, but not too warm. A pregnant woman's body temperature is usually higher than normal. Light as many candles as you can get your hands on, and that will fit in your bathroom without creating a fire hazard.

When she's comfortably in the water, read to her. Poetry, a novel, articles from a magazine, the ingredient label off the back of the ice cream carton. Just find something she'll enjoy and will help her to relax.

<u>(Week 14) What Can You Do?</u>

Materials:
• a functioning mouth
• the willingness to fulfill her requests

"My husband could have asked, 'What can I do for you to make you feel more comfortable?' Any sentence that started with, 'What can I do...' would have been very romantic and sweet during that time."
-Christine, California Business Owner

What to do:

It's simple. Remember, in romance, effort counts. Just ask what you can do for her: "What can I do to make you feel comfortable?", "What can I do to help you fall asleep?", "What can I do to help relieve your stress?", "What can I do to make your legs feel better?"

This is something you should start today and continue doing the rest of the pregnancy. Use it when you notice that your partner looks or acts uncomfortable or distressed. Step in and be her knight in shining armor, but be ready to do what she requests: a ten-minute shoulder rub, cooking dinner, or even a 2:00 a.m. run to the convenience store for rainbow sherbet.

If she knows you're looking out for her and that she can count on you, you'll have lifted a huge weight from her, which she'll appreciate long after Baby's arrival.

12

Trimester Two: The Easy Months

Just when you think you've got a handle on your partner's wants and needs, aversions and cravings, likes and dislikes, she goes and enters the second trimester. Once again, like every aspect of pregnancy, old rules, from trimester number one, are tossed out the window, and it's time to start fresh again.

There's good news, though. This trimester is called "the easy months" because most women report that during this time, they feel their best during pregnancy. The morning sickness portion of pregnancy is usually a thing of the past, while the swollen, and sometimes clumsy, stage has yet to cast its uncomfortable shadow.

Many men know that the middle portion of pregnancy is the time when women's energy levels rise, around the fourth month when the placenta is completed, and they show an increased appetite. But, most of us are pleasantly surprised to learn that there can also be an increase in sexual appetite. Many women find that with their emerging new bodies and the onset of motherhood, their libidos increase. And, almost as a gift from Mother Nature herself, with increased libido also comes increased vaginal lubrication.

So, there's a lot to look forward to during this second trimester, but realize that your partner may still feel fragile and vulnerable. Just because she's no longer vomiting after every meal and she's sleeping a bit less, doesn't mean other changes aren't taking place.

Your spouse may start to experience heartburn and/or constipation. Spider veins, varicose veins, and stretch marks are not uncommon as you enter the second trimester. And, around the fourth month her weight gain will start to become noticeable. She'll begin to "look pregnant". All of these changes may make some women feel unattractive. That, with the development of back, leg and hip pain, would cause any sane pregnant woman to desire some attention from her man.

Her hormone levels will start to stabilize around the fourth month. So, the weepiness and moodiness you may have noticed during the first three months may subside, but she'll most likely remain emotional and vulnerable for the rest of her pregnancy. She needs you now, as she will every step of this incredible journey. Enjoy.

(Week 15) Table for two

Materials:

- your best china
- your best silverware
- candles
- matches
- bouquet
- invitation
- your best crystal
- table cloth and napkins
- candleholders
- vase
- food

"I wish he'd cooked a surprise dinner for me with cloth napkins, candlelight, our nice china, and the works. A particularly nice touch would have been to serve bubble water in our nice crystal, which was collecting dust. This would have felt romantic because it would have seemed like one of our dates before we were married."
-Lynne, Associate Director

What to do:

A pregnant woman wants to be pampered every now and then, not because she's pregnant, but because she's your wife. Let her know that you two can still enjoy the things you did before pregnancy, or even before marriage.

You're probably already taking up slack by preparing more meals nowadays. And, with her increase in appetite, what better way to show your partner that you're thinking of her, than with a surprise four-course meal?

Pick a day this week. Send her an invitation to keep her calendar free for that evening. Rummage through your packed-away wedding gifts, and pull out your best, you know, the stuff she tells you she's saving for a special occasion. What's more special than an evening with the woman you love?

Stash aside the dinnerware, the silverware, including all three fork sizes, linen, candlesticks and candles. Then, you must prepare the meal. Make something special: lobster, a pasta dish, whatever she'll find appetizing. Don't forget the soup, salad, bread, beverages, and dessert. When you shop for your items, be sure to pick up a bouquet to put on the table, and garnishes, like parsley, for the plate.

(Week 16) To the Tea

Materials:
- tea
- hot water
- teacup
- spoon
- sweetener (optional)

"He made me tea."

-S. E., Teacher

What to do:
I know. It's so simple. Yet, it's tremendously effective. When she comes home sometime this week, ask her if she'd like some tea. Or, if you already know she'd appreciate it, make it for her as a surprise. If she responds favorably, make it a habit every now and then. I know a lot of pregnant women who wouldn't head off to bed without their cup of tea.

There are teas blended specifically for pregnancy. One many find effective is a combination of raspberry leaf, nettle, and alfalfa.

Raspberry leaf relaxes and strengthens the uterus for delivery. It also helps nausea. Nettle increases milk production and can reduce leg cramping. Alfalfa contains iron and calcium and may stimulate vitamin k in Mom.

Other teas include peppermint (which soothes upset tummies), meadowsweet (which is known as nature's Tums), and soothing chamomile. Before trying any new teas or herb, it's always best to run it by your doctor first.

<u>(Week 17) Pickles and Ice Cream</u>

Materials:
- car keys
- car
- sweat pants
- cash

"He went out one night specifically to buy me bologna for that one sandwich I had to make - I never eat bologna, but I really wanted one sandwich!"

-Thalia, Medical Transcriptionist

What to do:
The cravings may still make unannounced visits now and again. If Mom tells you she really could go for sardines and peanut butter and all you have stocked in the pantry is tuna and almond paste, be ready to head out to the corner store to fulfill her peculiar tastes.

For some reason, though, Mom won't call you from work to stop at the market on the way home. It's often a right-before-you-go-to-sleep craving. So, be willing to get out of bed without much fussing, throw on some sweat pants, and head out the door. It probably won't happen every night, especially at this stage in the pregnancy, and she'll appreciate you being there for her.

<u>(Week 18) Flower Power</u>

Materials:
• a bouquet of flowers
• a vase
• water
• an aspirin

"I wish he'd brought home flowers for me and put them in a vase before I got home. Just bringing home flowers is romantic, but the extra step of putting them in vases shows that a) he is trying to save me from having to do any extra work, and b) he is helping make our house a beautiful home."

-L. S., Age 35

What to do:
A surprise gift of flowers is always a welcome romantic gesture. They show your partner that she's on your mind, and, as L. S. said, they help to add beauty to your home.

This week come home with a bouquet for you partner. When she asks, "What's this for?" tell her it's to say "thank you" for carrying our baby."

Don't just give her the bouquet and expect her to peel the wrapping, clip the stems, find a vase, arrange the flowers, fill the vase with water and add a crushed aspirin so they will last longer. If you're giving her the flowers, don't make her work for them.

If you wanted to give your partner a string of pearls, you wouldn't come home one day with a bucket of oysters and some thread saying, "When you find one, string it through here. Hope you like them." So, don't do it with the flowers, either.

(Week 19) Trip the Light

Materials:
• loose pants
• comfortable shoes
• a credit card

"Take us dancing."

-R. H., Manager

What to do:
Yes, pregnant women love to dance, too. I can remember during the eighth month of my wife's second pregnancy, we were at a friend's wedding, and she was out on that dance floor with me, taking it easy, mind you, but dancing to her heart's content. Now, she was a bit on the larger side, and dips were certainly out of the question. But now, during week nineteen, is the perfect time to take your partner dancing. She's passed the nausea and fatigued phases and has yet to become so swollen and uncomfortable that tripping the light fantastic sounds too unappealing.

This week ask her out on a date. Suggest a night of dancing. She'll be thrilled that you asked and that you see her more than merely a pregnant woman, but still as the woman who can go out on the town and spend quality time with her man. Be sure, though, that she doesn't overexert herself, that the place you choose is a non-smoking establishment and that she's enjoying the music, dancing, and your company alcohol-free.

(Week 20) Say "Cheese"

Materials:
• camera
• film

• lingerie, a robe, your button-down shirt

"When I was about twenty weeks and started to feel like a baby whale, my husband took some photos of me in sexy underwear to show me how gorgeous he thought I was. I was still his wife and lover, not just a mother-to-be."
-S. F., Age 33

What to do:

Remember, during this second trimester women really start to show. They begin to look pregnant. People start to notice their changes, and many moms-to-be become self-conscious. They question their attractiveness and may need some sign of encouragement from the men they love.

This week tell her you've really been noticing how beautiful she's been looking lately. Let her know she's got a glow about her and you want to capture it on film. She may be reluctant at first, but be sure to let her know you're planning sexy, yet tasteful, photos.

To make her feel comfortable and beautiful, pick a location where she doesn't have to be self-conscious. If you have a private backyard or would like to use a room indoors, be sure that it's just the two of you. No neighbors. Send the kids to a movie. Also, play some music that will allow your partner to not only feel at ease, but to smile.

Try her in tasteful poses in her lingerie. You can also have her wearing a robe or even one of your button-down work shirts. Be sure to get some shots with the tummy exposed, because you want her to realize she's beautiful, not in spite of her growing mid-section, but that bump in her stomach is partly what is so attractive.

You can use props, too. Your partner holding a bud yet to blossom represents the growing child in her stomach. You can stage a shot of her reading one of her baby books in her robe, which is open enough to see her tummy. Or even a shot of her hand placed on her midsection can represent the anticipation of what's to come, and can be a beautiful and even sexy photo.

(Week 21) Surprise!

Materials:
• friends
• food
• music

"He threw me a surprise thirtieth birthday party because my plans for a girls' trip to Vegas were shot, due to pregnancy. That was verrry impressive. It really isn't like him to put such thought and effort into things like that. So, it was really wonderful."
-Brenda R., Mommy to Two

What to do:
It doesn't have to be a birthday party or even a party for a specific occasion. If you can't find something on the calendar, have a party anyway. But, make sure that it's a surprise.

You'll need to start arranging this a few weeks early. Pick a date and a place. You could choose the beach, your home, a restaurant, a friend's house. Then, make an invitation list. Choose people who will be fun. This is not a shower, so you're not obligated to invite great-aunts and her boss. Make sure you enlist the help of her friends. Hopefully they'll keep the secret, but more importantly, they can help you with the arrangements: food, gifts, decorations, etc...

When everyone yells, "Surprise!" she'll be stunned and will be sure to ask, "What's all this for?" Hug her. Tell her you love her. And, let her know you arranged this because you want to thank her for hanging in there the first half of the pregnancy.

(Week 22) Snakes, Snails, Sugar, and Spice

Materials:
• the ultrasound results

• a very trusting partner
• balloons, baby clothes, confetti, ribbon, anything that represents the sex of your baby

"My husband surprised me with the sex of our two children. We had the ultrasound performed and only he found out what we were going to have. With our first child, he threw me a baby shower where I found out what I was going to have by opening up presents and seeing the blue clothing. The second time around he filled up my car with balloons, ribbons, confetti, everything he could find that was blue, so that when I finished with my class at school and opened the door I'd know it was another boy. It was a great experience knowing that he was excited about our pregnancy and the way he informed me of the sex was romantic to me."
-Christina L, Age 21

What to do:

Yes, it's that time. Any day now, you and your spouse will be able to get your first glimpse at the new life you've created through the modern miracle known as the ultrasound. What an incredible time we live in, when we can share the visual image of our child with our partner even before birth. Some doctors now have the newest in baby-visioning, an ultrasound that projects a three-dimensional image of your child: facial features, body shape, you can even count fingers and toes.

No matter the type of ultrasound your doctor uses, she'll be able to determine Baby's sex at this stage in the game. Some couples want to know right away. Others want to be surprised. I can't be sure how many moms-to-be there are like Christina (above), but if you and your partner are adventuresome, you might consider his method of sex revealing.

Keep in mind, this may not be for every couple. But, if you'd like to know Baby's sex and Mom doesn't mind having that information revealed to her when she least expects it, then this week, when you attend the ultrasound appointment, be sure the doctor knows your plan as a couple. The doctor will inform you if you'll be having a boy or a girl. Then, the fun begins.

First, you'll have to keep your lips sealed. Can't let it slip. If you're a sleep-talker, wear a gag to bed. Next, pick a way and time to spring the news on your partner. Use Christina's husband's ideas: the baby shower and the car full of blue baby items. Or, come up with something on your own: a full page ad in the local paper, hire a skywriter, make a collage of pictures of little boys from magazines, serve a pink meal to announce the arrival of a girl: shrimp and salmon, pink lemonade, mashed potatoes with a dash of red food coloring.

If you can keep a secret and your partner is truly up for this, the way you present this surprise could truly be a memorable and romantic milestone in your relationship.

(Week 23) Chivalry Is Not Dead

Materials:
• heavy stuff
• a car or house with a door

"I would have liked to be treated more like I felt: fragile and delicate. Open doors, help me up, carry things."
-Jennifer, Full Time Mom

What to do:
Although many women feel their best during this time in their pregnancies, it doesn't mean we get to forget that they're still physically, hormonally, and emotionally unstable at times. Jennifer coined it nicely: "fragile and delicate."

If you're not already acting like her Prince Charming, her Superman, her knight in shining armor, it's time you step up this week and show her that you are a true gentleman. Open doors for her:

car, house, office, microwave oven, etc... Help her up from the sofa or floor. Remember her belly is growing. The ligaments in her hips may be sore due to stretching. And, carry things for her. She shouldn't be lifting heavy items, anyway. She's already carrying the weight of the baby, the retained water in her feet, the weight of her new placenta, 50% more blood, and a couple of sand-bags disguised as breasts. You carrying the groceries into the house might be the wise choice.

<u>(Week 24) Just Ask</u>

Materials:
• the wherewithal to think of her when you think of you
• a mouth in operational status

"During pregnancy, my husband always asked me if I needed anything when he got up to get something, so I didn't have to get up or go up or down stairs. It was very thoughtful."
-Cheryl P., Teacher

What to do:
When others ask us if they can help, if there's something they can do or if we need something, we feel looked out for, cared for, safe and secure. In essence, we feel loved. During pregnancy, not only are these acts kind and romantic, but they're extremely practical.

Mom may not be as fatigued as she was last trimester, but she may be a bit sore and uncomfortable. Starting this week, make a conscious effort to ask your partner if you can get her something or do something for her when you're up. You go to the kitchen for a snack, ask if she needs something: a piece of fruit, maybe a bowl of cereal. You head upstairs for a baseball cap, maybe she'd like it if you brought her book down from her nightstand. You go outside to the mailbox to see what bills you have to pay; it's possible she'd appreciate you getting the cell phone she left in the car.

You won't know unless you ask. It's simple. Tell her where you're going and ask if she needs something: "I'm going upstairs. Do you need anything while I'm there?" This display of caring will make the love of your life feel looked after, and physically she'll feel stronger and have more energy because you thought of her when you were thinking of yourself.

(Week 25) It's On Me

Materials:
• credit card, checkbook, cash, or gift certificate

"(My husband) encouraged me to go shopping and buy nice things to wear and always made me feel beautiful."
                              -Rebecca, New Mom From Britain

What to do:
Now that your partner is looking pregnant, she may be feeling a bit self-conscious about her appearance. Although some women's confidence blossoms during pregnancy, many feel that they are no longer attractive to their partners. Also, some women associate maternity clothes with frumpy muumuus of the '70's.

This week show your partner that she's still beautiful with her changing body. Hand her the credit card, the checkbook, cold hard cash, or a gift certificate to a shop that sells fashionable maternity wear. You might be surprised by the array of up-to-date apparel now being made exclusively for pregnant women. Encourage your partner to get one of these cute, contemporary outfits. They're even making sexy cocktail dresses and lingerie for moms-to-be. If you encourage your partner to get something to make her feel attractive, she will feel attractive. When she feels attractive, her confidence and self-esteem climb, and she becomes even more appealing. It becomes an ongoing cycle of beauty, self-confidence and romance.

<u>(Week 26) Shoot for Comfort</u>

Materials:
• Victoria's Secret catalog
• credit card

"Buy her comfy PJ's."

-Leon Scott Baxter, Romance Guru

What to do:
Okay, so this idea didn't come from the wonderful women who've been so kind to help me with this book. It's advice from me, but it's been backed by woman after woman.

I have a website (CouplesCommittedToLove.com) where I offer a daily romantic tip. One tip is for the fellas to buy their spouses comfy flannel pajamas, rather than skimpy sexy ones. The reason: the flannel ones feel better, so women will wear them more often. When they wear them they feel good, and feeling good can lead to feeling sexy. When she's feeling sexy, the flannel pajamas come off quicker.

Then, pregnant women told me that I should offer dads-to-be the "comfy PJ's" advice. It's not so much to get her out of her pajamas when she's pregnant, but to make her feel good and comfy.

This week as your wife's belly expands another inch or two, you may notice elastic lines left on her midsection in the morning from her tight sleeping garments. Pull out the Victoria's Secret catalog, skip the skimpy PJ's and ask her to pick out some comfortable sleeping apparel. She'll love being able to shop on your dime. But, more importantly, she knows you're thinking of her and understanding her needs.

I remember when my wife got her huge, roomy, not-so-sexy, blue, flannel pajamas during her second pregnancy, She'd crack a smile just by putting them on. If I even mentioned pajamas, a sparkle came to her eye. I couldn't get her out of the things until noon on weekends. She loved them, not only because they felt so nice, but also because they represented security and love.

(Week 27) Can You Hear Me Now?

Materials:
• a clear throat
• a book (optional)

"I think the most romantic thing my husband does is talk to the baby. He does it every night. He wants her to hear his voice as much as possible. He holds small conversations with her and sometimes reads to her."

-Lindsay, Artist

What to do:
Baby's hearing starts developing the fifth month of pregnancy, and there's a good chance he can hear what's going on outside the womb during the sixth month.

So, right around now is the time to start getting your child used to your voice. Baby hears Mom talking all day: at work, with you, on the phone, in the grocery store, etc... But you'll need to make an effort to have Baby know Dad's sound.

Starting this week make a point to talk to the bulge whenever you can. But, more importantly, start a ritual, same time everyday, to either read a book to your wife's tummy, tell it about your day at work, or even sing it a song or two. And, every time you talk, rub Mom's tummy. Not only will Mom feel soothed by the gentle strokes on her abdomen, but Baby will be alerted to your voice through touch, also.

Why is this romantic to your partner? Anything you do to show her that you are caring for the baby she's carrying lets her know that you will be a terrific dad. She'll feel comfortable and safe with this knowledge. Your actions become endearing to her, serotonin levels increase and Mom-to-be feels romanced.

13

Trimester Three: The Uncomfortable Months

It's coming down to the wire. Remember when that due date the doctor told you so many months ago seemed forever away? Now, there's a light at the end of this tunnel. For many couples this last trimester is when reality sets in. It's really going to happen. You're going to be parents.

What a journey it's been. By the end of this trimester, many men see their partners in a new light. You may respect your spouse in ways you never could have imagined before you embarked upon this experience. You may have seen a strength and confidence in her that only pregnancy could have brought to the surface.

That strength and confidence can be tested these last three months. They're called the "uncomfortable months" because along with the anxiety and eagerness to finally meet Baby, Mom's tummy really starts to bulge. She may feel awkward and clumsy. She may experience varicose veins and hemorrhoids, as well as swollen feet and hands.

Because of her increasing size, your partner may experience discomfort in her neck and lower back, which can lead to difficulty sleeping at night. And, the pressure on her bladder will inevitably send her to the ladies' room more times in a day that you care to count.

She may suffer from heartburn or indigestion. Because of her increased temperature, a normally comfortable day to you may leave her perspiring profusely. All this, including possible sciatica (the inflammation of the sciatic nerve, resulting in pain from the lower back down the legs), Braxton-Hicks, which are uterine contractions preparing Mom's body for delivery, and Baby playing soccer with her bladder throughout the day help explain why many women experience a dramatic decrease in sexual desire during the third trimester.

But, all is not lost. Romance can still rise above the swollen, aching, insomniatic, clumsy, and anxious ashes of the third trimester, as long as you make the appropriate changes.

During the final leg of this procreation relay, Mom-to-be needs to relax. She'll find relief in your pampering, allowing her to rest, putting her feet up on pillows, massaging her back and feet and performing effleurage. There's never a time when someone does not want to be cared for or made to feel special. Therefore, there's never a time when we don't want to be romanced.

(Week 28) A Good Laugh

Materials:
• the Sunday paper
• construction paper
• glue
• staples
• a marker

"(My husband) put together a little book called, 'Ma-Ma-2B' out of comic strips that had something to do with pregnancy or babies. He spent nine months collecting them and presented the book to me toward the end of my pregnancy. It showed that he really cared about all the changes I was going through, and took the time to make something that we could enjoy and laugh at together for many years to come."

-Mary, Kindergarten Teacher

What to do:
Those folks who put together the comics for the newspaper certainly have mastered the art of allowing us to find humor in our mundane discomforts, from getting stuck in traffic to losing a sock in

the dryer. They allow us to laugh at ourselves without making us feel as though we're the butt of the joke.

If you keep your eyes peeled, you'll find that many of the comics deal with pregnancy, childbirth, and being parents. As parents-to-be we can see ourselves in these colorful panels: picking the baby's name, dealing with Mom's mood swings or food cravings, assembling the crib, or large breasts too tender to be touched.

Start collecting these comics that speak to you, that you'll appreciate, that your spouse will relate to her pregnancy. When you've got a decent collection, cut them out, glue them to construction paper, and staple together in a book format. If you have enough, you could even arrange the comic strips into sections: Morning Sickness, Delivery, New Parents, etc... Then, slap together a cover, maybe a photo of your hand on her belly or the two of you while she's pregnant, put a title on it, and present it to her when she's uncomfortable, hot, bothered and tired. Laughter can fix almost anything.

(Week 29) Sexy Mama

Materials:
• a big mouth

"He told me how sexy I looked even with a big tummy."
-Ellie, Age 40

What to do:
As you know, telling your partner that she's beautiful is crucial for her self-esteem during pregnancy. But, now, not only may she feel unattractive, she also may not feel very sexy. So, let her know that you think she is.

Just because you may no longer be having intercourse as much as you used to, if at all, doesn't mean that she's not sexy. Tell her about her glow. Let her know she's beautiful. Mention how sexy her tummy is and how her breasts are enticing. Letting your partner know this late in pregnancy that she's not only a baby-cocoon, but an alluring woman, will make her smile and bring a warmth to her heart.

(Week 30) Just One More Article

Materials:
• pregnancy and parenting magazines and books

"He read more parenting books than I did."
                                    -J. H., 27 Year-Old Teacher

What to do:
There are more books in your local bookstore about parenting and pregnancy than you can read during a nine-month pregnancy, even if you went without sleep, food or using the bathroom. There are also terrific magazines available on pregnancy and parenting.

Read some! Good chance your partner has some lying around. Find out what's going on with your wife's body. Learn about the development of your baby. Look into what it takes to be a good parent. When you start to read these books and articles, and you realize that they apply to you, your partner, and your baby, the fascination is immeasurable. You won't be able to put down the pages.

You'll find yourself spewing facts: "Did you know the baby is growing fingernails now?", "That line is called the Linea Negra, and will stick around after the baby's born", "I read that newborns can't distinguish between night and day." You may or may not enlighten your partner, but she'll definitely find your effort and enthusiasm endearing.

(Week 31) Fluff It Up

Materials:
• pillows, lots of pillows

"He would make a pillow bed for my naps."
                                    -Jenna, From California

What to do:
When Mom sleeps at this stage in her pregnancy, she can't lay on her stomach because her bulge gets in the way. She shouldn't sleep on her back because in this position her uterus partially blocks the vena cava, the baby's main blood source. Her only option: sleeping on her side. By the way, doctors recommend sleeping on the left side because many women have asymmetrical uteruses that lean to the right, putting pressure on the vena cava when they lie on the right.

So, make this position as comfortable as you can for her. Childbirth expert, Tracy Schmidt, instructs men to construct a "pillow nest" for their pregnant partners. You'll need six or more pillows, and the idea is to not allow any part of her body to rest on any other part of her body. You'll place a pillow under her head, one between her knees. One may support her tummy while another supports her back. Through a series of maneuvering and pillow-placement, Mom will feel cozy and comfy in her nest of pillows.

If you don't have the time, or own stock in a pillow company, you can still take a few and place them around, and under, Mom-to-be before she naps or goes to sleep for the night. She'll feel loved, will sleep easier, and will feel better rested in the morning.

For those of you who would like to offer more than the standard down pillow, a variety of pillows have been created solely for the sleeping comfort of pregnant women, including wedge-shaped pillows that can offer the "nest" feel. One behind your partner's back and one under her tummy will keep her secure and comfy. Check out maternity shops and stores online for more ideas.

(Week 32) A Little Mold Never Hurt Anyone

Materials:
• torso mold kit
• a naked, pregnant woman

"Last night, we made a plaster mold of my wife's belly. At the baby shower we plan on having our guests sign it."
-J. G., First-Time Dad-To-Be

What to do:
It's a craze that's catching on, immortalizing the glorious roundness of your pregnant partner's torso. This week look into getting your hands on one of these kits. They're listed online from $20 on up to over $100. They claim to be easy to use and many guarantee quality.

The whole process of plastering your partner's chest and tummy can be a fun experience. Then, having a plaster copy of her for memory's sake, so Baby can see how Mommy looked when he was in her tummy, or for guests to sign at the baby shower makes the mold worth trying.

(Week 33) Your Slippers, Madame

Materials:
• bathtub
• bathrobe
• slippers
• candles
• soothing music
• book or magazine
• fluffy towels
• sparkling juice, tea, or some other beverage

"Brad would have a warm bath ready for me when I came home from work. My bathrobe, slippers, book, and sparkling juice would all be arranged. What a homecoming!"

-Heather, Fourth Grade Teacher

What to do:

With her swollen ankles, enflamed sciatic nerve, and lower back pain, what a relief it would be for your partner to come home this week to find a mini-evening-at-the-spa in her own home.

At least once this week while your wife is at work or has gone out on an errand, get the bathroom prepared for her. Pull out her bathrobe and slippers. If she doesn't have any, or they're getting on the shabby side, buy her some new ones. She can bring them along with her to the hospital for the delivery. Light all sorts of candles and have relaxing music playing for her. Be sure her current novel or a few magazines are stacked alongside the tub for her reading pleasure. And, don't forget to have a sparkling fruit juice, cup of tea, or some other relaxing, non-alcoholic, non-soft drink beverage available for her to whet her palate.

Help your partner in the tub. Whisk her clothes away to the hamper. Then, leave her alone if she needs solitude, or sit by the tub and gently rub her tummy if she requests your company. When it's time for your partner to exit the bath, be sure you're there with a helping hand. That big tummy can really cause havoc on a woman's center of gravity. As she steps out of the tub, wrap her in a warm, fluffy towel. Help to dry her, and drape her robe over her. Give your partner a kiss and tell her you're in love with her.

(Week 34) Capture Her Image

Materials:
• charcoal, pencil, markers, paint, or crayons
• paper or canvas

• (optional) eraser, paintbrush, Liquid Paper

"He drew a charcoal sketch of me in my full ninth month glory. It hangs now in our bedroom."

-Melissa, New Mom

What to do:
Remember, many almost-moms are unhappy with the way their bodies transform during pregnancy, especially in these later weeks. Your taking interest in not only your partner, but especially in her changing body, lets Mom-to-be know that the changes are not only okay, but beautiful.

This week, ask her if she'll pose for you as you attempt to capture her image via charcoal, pencil, markers, or even crayon. If you have some artistic ability, great. You'll have no trouble with this. But, if you're like the majority of dads-to-be, you're more of a Michael Moore than a Michelangelo.

Don't worry, though. If your artistic talents leave something to be desired, still give it a go. You two will have such a blast just playing artist and model. Be sure she doesn't see your piece of art until it's complete. And, if the only brush you've ever held is one with Colgate at the end, don't try to make your piece realistic. Go the Picasso route; draw the hair, some lips, an eye and a big belly. Or, do something symbolic: a budding flower or a nest with a sparrow's egg.

The piece of art will be kept, not necessarily for what you've created on the canvas, but as a reminder of the fun you two shared making it.

(Week 35) Is It Ripe?

Materials:
• bulbous fruit: oranges, melons, and peaches

"During my second pregnancy, every week he'd bring home fruit that looked like pregnant women: watermelons, cantaloupe, fuzzy peaches. He'd tell me, 'It reminded me of you.' It was romantic because it was acknowledgment of my pregnancy and my changing body. It was really sweet."

-Jill D., Mid-Wife

What to do:

What a creative and loving way for a man to let his pregnant partner know that she's on his mind. This week, while you're at the grocery store or the local produce stand, look for fruit that reflects the fullness of your partner. Bring it home, and tell her it reminded you of her when you saw it.

Knowing that you are able to see her in other objects tells your partner that she's on the forefront of your mind and that this pregnancy is important to you. But, most of all, it lets her know that *she's* important to you. And, that's really the fruit of the tree of romance.

(Week 36) Did You See That?

Materials:
• floor, couch, or bed
• pregnant woman wearing a shirt or blouse

"We'd sit on the couch and he'd want my shirt up so he could check out the baby. It made the changes in my body seem sexy, instead of grotesque."

-Cathi S., 32 Year-Old Mother of two

What to do:

No doubt, there are times that your partner's stomach will appear imbalanced. The baby will be smooshed up on one side, or maybe there'll be a huge uneven bulge sticking out from one part. Then, if you wait long enough, the bulge moves. The baby may kick or roll to the other side. It may be jerky or roll like a wave.

These lumps and bumps are out of Mom's control and can seem like a scene from a sci-fi movie. Or, the movement and bulges can be looked at as a beautiful opportunity to see life during its final stages before emerging into our world.

This week when Mom says, "I felt it kick," or "Look at this bulge," sit her down and pull up her shirt. Marvel at the life below her skin. Rub her stomach and feel your baby. Smile at Mom when you can feel in move. Find beauty in your wife. Find beauty in life.

(Week 37) Spa Evening

Materials:

• bubble bath	• soothing CD
• pumice stone	• rose petals
• foot massage lotion	• cotton balls
• chocolates	• a beverage
• toe nail polish	• her robe

"(My husband) created a 'spa evening' for me for our anniversary including a wonderful pedicure. He bought all the stuff. What a treat! Dark chocolates and an hour-long foot treatment: scrub, massage, hot soak, more massage, and lovely red toenails!."
-Tracy, Oldest Child - 22/ Youngest - 8

What to do:

For most women it's such a treat to receive the gift of a day at the spa. But, if you don't have the finances for it, there are no spas nearby, or you'd just rather be more involved personally, you can create "Spa de la Casa" (The Home Spa). Although you may have no experience with doling out the spa treatment, your enthusiasm and effort can really make the experience a treat for your partner.

You can offer to pamper your partner for an anniversary or for another special occasion: birthday, Mother's day, Valentine's Day. Or, you can just surprise her this week for no apparent reason other than you want to relax and please her.

First, draw a warm bath for your pregnant partner. You can make it a bubble bath or float rose petals from your local florist on the water. As always, candles and soothing music can add to the ambiance.

As she soaks, prepare for her pedicure. Get some towels ready. Fluff some pillows. Have a cup of tea, a glass of water with a lemon twist, or a saucer of chocolates within her reach. Pull out your pumice stone, massage oil, and toenail polish.

When your pedicure area is ready, help your partner from the tub. Pat her dry with towels, and drape her in her robe. Walk her to your pedicure station where you'll set her comfortably on the fluffed pillows. Show your partner the refreshments. And, with her tootsies over a towel, begin rubbing the pumice stone on the rough part of her feet. All that weight on her dogs can make them rough and calloused.

When you've got them soft again, work that foot lotion on her feet. Gently rub her heels and arches and even between her toes being sure her feet are always elevated to relieve the edema. When you've completed the foot rub, stick some cotton balls between her toes and start painting those nails.

Many women neglect foot care during these last weeks of pregnancy because they're just too difficult to reach. Your care and attention to her feet and the rest of her body will demonstrate to your partner how very much you love her.

<u>(Week 38) Fend For Yourself</u>

Materials:
• a mouth with a zipper on the lips

"(My husband) did not put pressure on me to keep the house clean, have the cupboards full of food, have sex, etc... If I wanted to lay on the couch all day, that was okay with him. That showed how much he cared and loved me, which is always romantic."

-Christine M., (34), First Time Mom

What to do:

This week, it sounds pretty simple: think before you speak. In all relationships, we develop roles, or jobs, if you will; one person mows the lawn, the other balances the checkbook. One does the shopping, the other feeds the cats. One fills the ice trays, the other puts out the trash.

As the delivery date quickly approaches, Mom-to-be may be finding it difficult to keep up with her responsibilities. She knows this. She realizes that you're out of paper towels and that the answering machine messages haven't been cleared. There's no need to remind her. She's not choosing to neglect her duties out of laziness. She's working terribly hard with that child in her belly.

So, make it a point to avoid adding more pressure or stress on your partner. If you see something needs to be done, instead of telling her she needs to water the plants, pick up the watering can and do it for her. If you're not sure how to do something, ask. Don't make her feel guilty, "I'm doing your job because you're too tired." Just ask without any malice. Avoid putting her on the defensive: "Where do you keep the fabric softener?" She'll know immediately that you're stepping in and stepping up to fill her shoes, and she'll appreciate it more than you'll know.

(Week 39) She's Got Your Nose

Materials:
• old photos of you and your partner as babies

"On our anniversary (when I was nine-plus months pregnant), after an amazing meal at a very intimate restaurant, my husband suggested we take our own baby albums to my parent's house to dream about our future little one's possible features."
-Heather, Age 33

What to do:

You can't help but wonder: "Will she have my eyes?" or "Do you think she'll have your dimple?" When you look in the mirror, don't you imagine that nose on a baby? Well, your partner's wondering it, too.

What a fun way to bring the two of you closer while focusing on your little one this week. Get ahold of both your and your partner's baby photos. You may need to do a bit of legwork; call her folks, stop by your parents' attic.

Then, make an evening of it. Spread the pictures all over the floor and look at the features the two of you were born with. Have any stuck? Could these be the ones that Baby will be born with? What did you both have in common as babies? Chubby cheeks? A head full of hair? Does that mean that Baby will have these, too?

What features were contradictory between the two of you? Ears flat against her head, sticking out on yours? Round eyes on you, oval eyes on her? Which will be dominant in the baby?

Play with different combinations. Talk to your partner about her best features. Tell her what you hope the baby gets of hers.

I remember when my wife and I discussed our baby's facial features. We were both in agreement and crossing our fingers that she did not get my wife's nose nor my ears. It was fine to laugh at ourselves and fun to point out our partners' beauty. An activity like this not only allows the two of you to dream about your future, but to live in your present.

(Week 40) Cutting It Close

Materials:
• bowl
• warm water
• razor
• shaving cream

"When I went into labor on each of my three pregnancies, my husband popped out of bed, ran and made me toast and a cup of tea and brought a big warm bowl of water, the razor, and the shaving cream to the couch and shaved my legs before we went to the hospital. This was always a moment cherished for me, because he knew that I hadn't even been able to see my legs for three months!"
-Rachael S., Age 34

What to do:
It doesn't even cross many men's minds that one of pregnancy's inconveniences is the difficult job of leg shaving. Men don't think about it because men don't shave their legs. Many women feel uncomfortable or unkempt with stubbly legs. When your partner goes into labor, she'll be exposing herself physically and emotionally to strangers. But, if she has some control over her appearance, at least part of her world during this chaotic experience will be her own.

For most women, when they start labor, there is plenty of time before having to rush to the hospital. You can drop the kids off at Grandma's. You can both shower. There should be time to call the in-laws and even make and eat a meal.

So, this week, if this is the big one, when she says it's time to go, ask if she'd like her legs shaved. If she says yes, fill a bowl full of water, lather her legs like you would your chin, and shave in long smooth strokes. Your heart may be pounding like it wants to escape, knowing that your baby will soon arrive, but keep a steady hand. Odds are Baby won't arrive for a few more hours.

Your partner will remember this as one of the final acts of love you performed before your newest addition sprang into your life. Memories of love and romance during her pregnancy will be the foundation of the love and romance you two will continue to foster during your relationship long after Baby arrives.

14

Your Journey Has Only Begun

You started this journey through a physical manifestation of love. You and your partner came together to create another person to share your lives with, to share your love with. Love and romance ignited this adventure. So, it's only appropriate that this adventure be filled with love and romance.

An acquaintance of mine recently asked me why it's so important to keep romance alive during pregnancy. There's the obvious response: a romanced partner is a happy partner; when she's happy she's experiencing a healthier pregnancy, and when romance is abundant in a relationship, that relationship is abundant with warmth and security.

But, more importantly, keeping romance alive during pregnancy sets the groundwork for the long haul. If the two of you are already sharing the benefits of romance while she's carrying your child, you'll be more likely to continue down romance's path after Baby arrives.

I can't seem to get a straight answer, but I've heard it was Abraham Lincoln, David O. McKay, and even Theodore Hesburgh who once said, "The most important thing a father can do for his children is to love their mother." No matter who first uttered these words, they rang true when they were spoken, and their echoes resonate truth today. Your love for your partner is crucial to your family's stability. It's the spark that initially ignited this family and will be the foundation that keeps it solid and grounded.

The romance you bestow on your partner during pregnancy will lead to the romance you bestow upon her during the newborn weeks, the baby months, and the toddler years. That romance will keep your family happy and alive and grinning. It will teach love to your children while strengthening the bonds with your partner. Your romance teaches everyone who's paying attention that sharing is okay, that kindness is painless, that respect is crucial. Your children will learn so much about life through the love and romance you offer their mother. Your children will not only survive, but they will excel in social settings, at school, and eventually in romantic relationships of their own.

It all starts now, even before Baby arrives. Mom wants to know that romance will always be a part of your relationship, even during life's big changes. Romance should never take a vacation from your relationship, because everyday your partner needs to know she's important, she's special, and she's cared for, by you, the father of her child. The time and effort you put forth during these nine months are investments that will reap dividends for a lifetime.

The mother of your child is your cherished diamond in a world filled with granite and quartz. Treat her as such.

"I found it very sexy when my husband treated me with the same care and consideration he would have used with a precious gem."
-J. C., Mom

Congratulations.

Be A Part Of Our Books

A book such as this would have been virtually impossible without the help of others who'd actually been through the experience of pregnancy. The quotes from all of the moms, new moms, moms-to-be and dads brought my theoretical romantic ideas to a practical reality.

Now that you've experienced pregnancy and are soon-to-be parents, we'd love know what you thought of *A Labor With Love*. We'd also like to share your experiences with other new parents and parents-to-be through updated versions of *A Labor With Love* as well as upcoming books. We want to know what you found romantic during pregnancy and why. What would have been romantic? Why?

Future books are in the works covering romance for couples during the newborn weeks, the baby months, and the toddler years. We'd love to hear from both Mom and Dad:
- What worked for you in the romance area?
- What were the biggest obstacles?
- What was the most romantic thing?
- What would have been romantic?

We always want to know why and how. Also, tell us the age of the baby (newborn, baby, toddler) so we may determine in which book to use your quote.

We'd love to know about you, also:
- Name
- Male/ Female
- Age
- Where you were raised
- Where you currently reside
- Occupation
- How many children you have, their ages and sex

Email the information to Leon Scott Baxter at info@CouplesCommittedToLove.com. If you'd like us to notify you if your quote is used, enclose your contact information: address, email, and/or phone.

Finally enclose a brief release so that we may use your quote: "I give to Leon Scott Baxter the right to reprint any portion of the enclosed experience in future books or articles."

If there are any parts of the aforementioned that you do not feel comfortable including, feel free to exclude them. The more you include, though, the easier it will be for us to use, but we don't want you to feel uncomfortable.

We thank you for your interest. Without help from people like you, these books could never be made.

BIBLIOGRAPHY

Baxter, Leon Scott. *Out of the Doghouse*. Santa Barbara: Lewski Books, 2003.

Chapman, Gary. *The Five Love Languages*. Chicago: Northfield Publishing, 1992.

Gray, John. *The Mars & Venus Diet & Exercise Solution*. New York: St. Martin's Press, 2003.

Jonas, Barbara & Michael. *The Book of Love, Laughter and Romance*. San Francisco: Games Partnership Ltd., Inc., 1994.

Murkoff, Heidi. *What to Expect When You're Expecting*. Workman Publishing, 2002.

Osbourne-Sheets, Carole. *Pre and Perinatal Massage Therapy*. Body Therapy Associates, 1998.

Wooden, John. *Wooden*. McGraw-Hill, 1997.

Leon Scott Baxter is not a doctor, medical practitioner, nor holds a degree in medicine. Neither the author, nor the book, *A Labor With Love*, claim to be a substitute for expert medical or professional advice of any kind. Be sure to check with a physician before implementing any change in exercise, diet, or lifestyle. Each woman is unique, and each pregnancy is different.